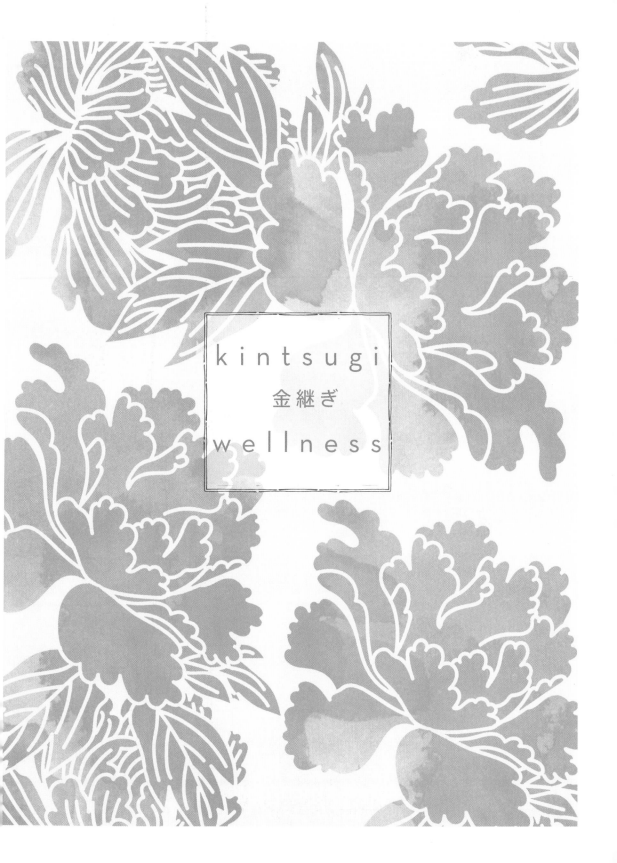

kintsugi

金継ぎ

wellness

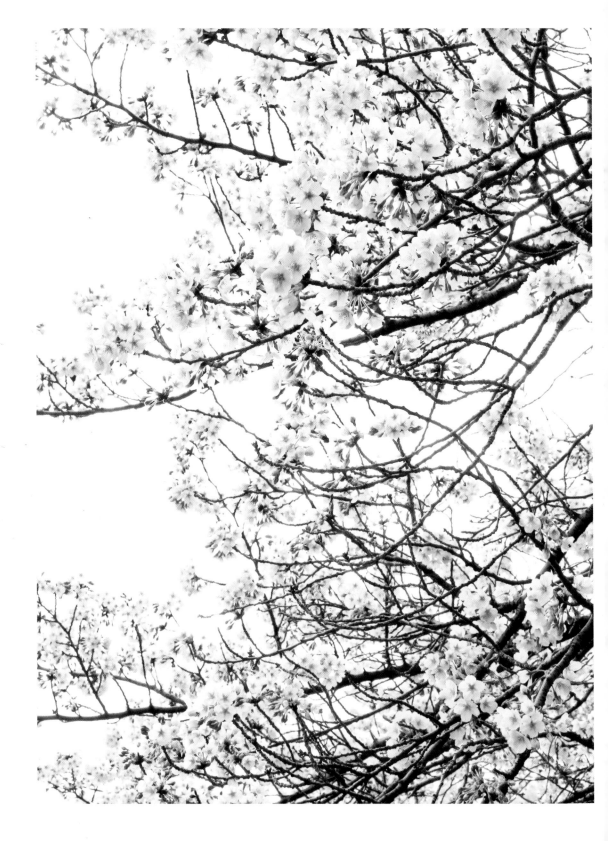

also by candice kumai

Clean Green Eats

Clean Green Drinks

Cook Yourself Sexy

Pretty Delicious

Cook Yourself Thin

the

japanese art

of nourishing

mind, body,

and spirit

kintsugi

金継ぎ

wellness

candice kumai

作者 / 撮影者 キャンディス 熊井

photographs by candice kumai

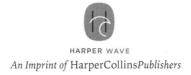

HARPER WAVE

An Imprint of **HarperCollins***Publishers*

おばあちゃん
我が家の長である祖母へ
あなたの生涯を誇りに
思い，祝い
あなたと日本の方々に
敬意を込めて
この本を捧げます。
深い感謝を込めて
引き継いでいきます。

Baachan,

Our family's Matriarch:
To honor and celebrate your life.
This book is an homage to you
& to the people of Japan.
We recieve your traditions & culture
with deep gratitude.

X. Caudill 熊井

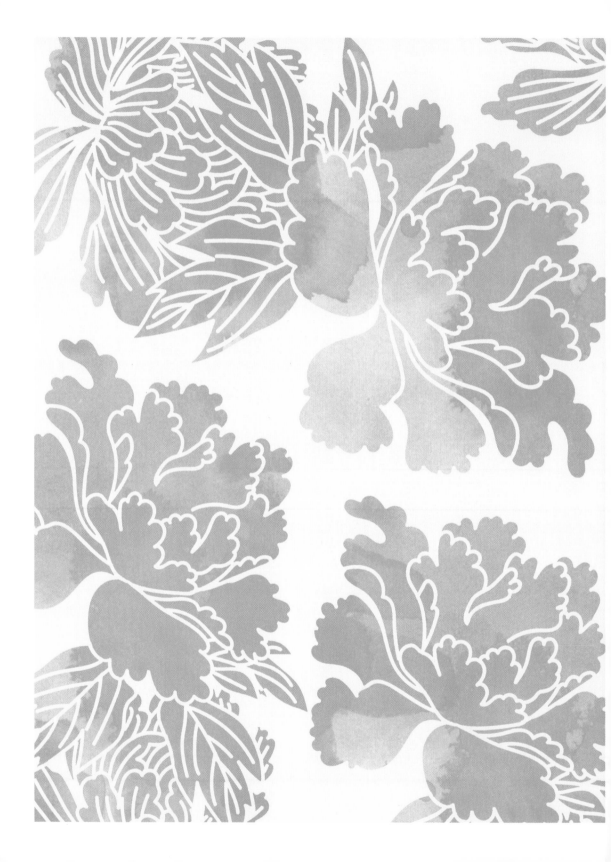

contents

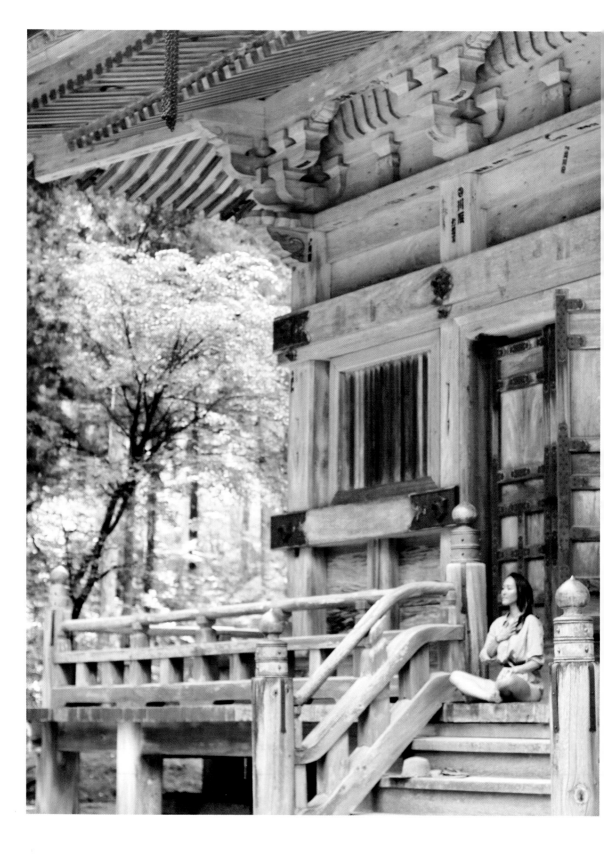

introduction

IT'S TAKEN ME THIRTY-PLUS YEARS TO WRITE THIS BOOK. Not because I didn't want to write it—the truth is, I've always wanted to write it—but I was very afraid of putting words on the page. After all, the prospect was intimidating. Japanese culture is largely focused on intricate detail, precision, and preparation. I never felt like I was "good enough" or "ready enough" to write a book about the cultural traditions I grew up with and the philosophies that have shaped my life and career.

I decided that the only way I would ever feel ready, or qualified, to write on this topic was to go back to my mother's ancestral home in Japan. To spend time visiting with all the family members whom I don't see often enough, to taste the flavors of Japan, to observe its traditions and rituals, to feel a part of its rhythms and its pulse. And so, a few years ago, I bought a ticket, packed my bags, and headed east.

I've explored Japan many times since I was five, but I knew from the moment I arrived that this trip would be different. From the moment the wheels of the plane touched down, I felt like I was home. I told myself to be brave, to open myself up to this opportunity, and to learn all that could be learned. Truth be told, I was fresh off a breakup and my heart was hurting. My mind felt foggy. My body was tired. I felt broken, and I secretly hoped that this journey would help to heal me.

Over the course of ten trips over the past few years, I experienced Japan during all four seasons. In the spring, I explored *hanami* (flower viewing) during the cherry blossom festival, and studied matcha tea ceremony with my great-aunt Takuko in Southern Japan. During the summer, I cooked homemade Japanese meals with my cousins in Tokyo and stayed with the monks in the mountains of Kōyasan. During the fall, I hiked the holy temples of Shikoku Island and learned how to cook with a Japanese *washoku* teacher back in Tokyo. In the winter, I drank sake with my friends in Niigata, ate delicious *nabe* hot pots in Matsuyama, and visited my favorite *onsen* baths in the Iya Valley. Japan experiences all four seasons, and the Japanese adapt to and appreciate all of them—the rain, the snow, the storms—whatever nature brings.

One day, I was in Kyoto, observing a *kintsugi* master, Tsuyoshi-san, at work in his home studio. He reminded me of my grandfather (an Impressionist painter), with his wisdom, artistic character, and massive amount of talent. Carefully, he sealed the pieces of broken pottery until they were whole again and painted the cracks with gold. As I watched this talented man put his energy and soul into bringing shattered vessels back to life, it hit me: kintsugi is the self-care we all need and deserve.

Kintsugi is applied to vessels that are not just broken, but beloved. The gold that seals the cracks is applied with an artist's care and devotion. The finished product is more beautiful than it was before. We deserve this too! And we shouldn't have to wait until we feel broken to give ourselves this gift.

It is through a process of self-care and self-acceptance that we can heal, flourish, and grow. My journey taught me so much, and, in the end, I left Japan feeling healed in mind, body, and spirit. My experience of learning how to put myself back together made me stronger, tougher, and more resilient.

As I was writing this book, I talked to my girlfriends and heard so many

Kōyasan, Japan: We can learn so much from the monks, admiring their tenacity, poise, and devotion.

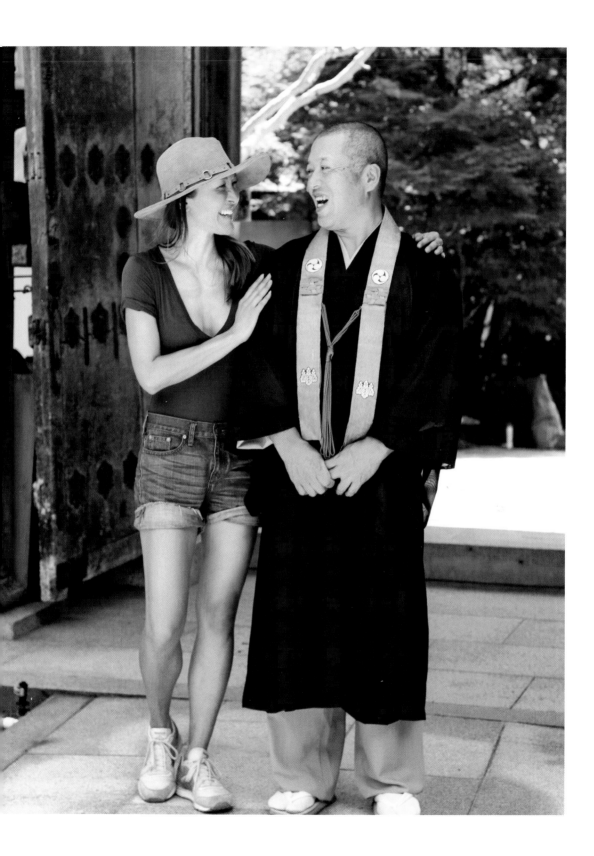

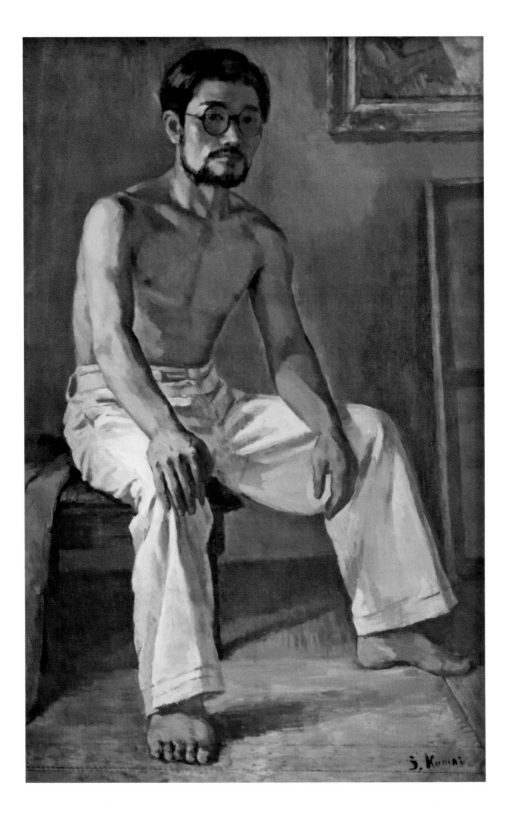

similar stories. I realized that too many of us feel broken or damaged—or simply not good enough—too much of the time. We're so busy being hard on ourselves that it's easy to lose sight of the fact that we are also deserving of the self-care it takes to maintain our health and our happiness. Golden repair celebrates our imperfections. It teaches us that we are more beautiful for our flaws, our battle scars, our lessons learned.

The philosophies of Japanese life are the guiding force of this book. I've organized them into four parts: Strengthen, Nourish, Lifestyle, and Heart. In each of these sections, you will find some of the simple rituals that helped heal me. In Japan, rituals are an important part of everyday life. These practices are prompts that remind you of what's important, and ground you in the present while honoring the past.

It is my hope that this book will offer you the golden repair you need to feel whole, vibrant, happy, and healthy. I'm excited to share my heritage, my family's traditions, and my heart.

体に 気 をつけて ください!

Karada ni ki o tsukete kudasai! Please take care of yourself,

キャンディス 熊井

Candice Kumai

My grandfather's self portrait: Jun Kumai's artwork is the lifeline to our family's artistry. He was a rebel before his time and a pioneer in his field. He traveled the world painting from the 1970s to the 1980s. He had a deep and profound love for Europe. A true *shokunin*.

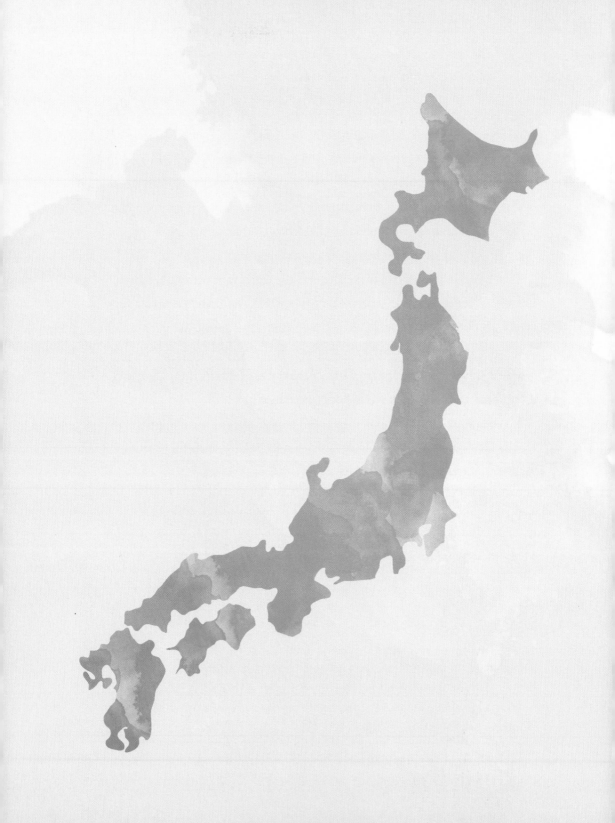

strengthen

jōbunisuru

丈夫にする，じょうぶにする/

genkizukeru

元気づける，げんきづける

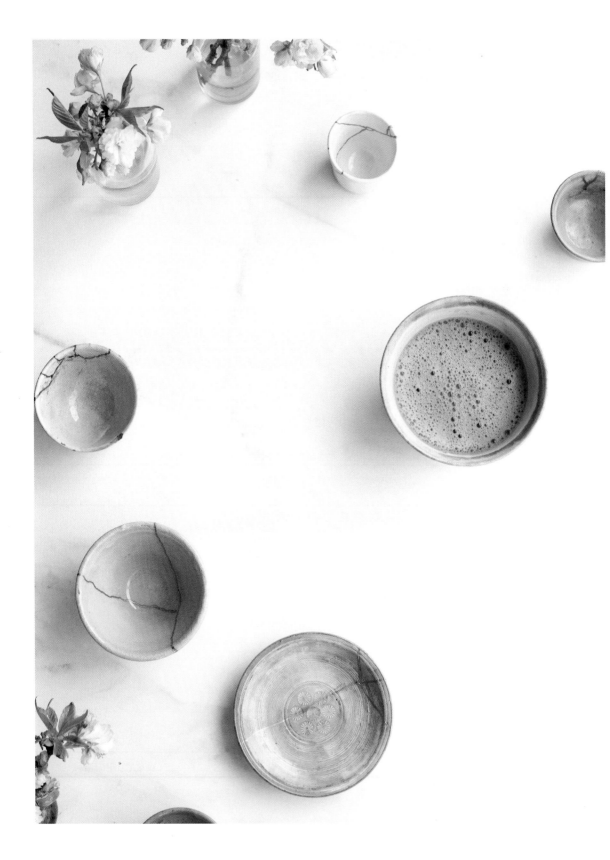

kintsugi

金継ぎ, きんつぎ

(keen tsu gee)

the japanese
art of
golden repair

Kɪɴᴛsᴜɢɪ, 金継ぎ,きんつぎ (keen tsu gee), translated from Japanese kanji meaning:

> 金—gold
> 継—repair, inherit, succeed, continue

Kɪɴᴛsᴜɢɪ ɪs ᴍʏ ʜᴇᴀʀᴛ. It is my life's anthem.

Kintsugi made me who I am today.

The practice of kintsugi—repairing broken vessels by sealing the cracks with lacquer and carefully dusting them with gold powder—is a remarkable art. The Japanese believe the golden cracks make the pieces even more precious and valuable.

It's beautiful to think of this practice as a metaphor for your life, to see the broken, difficult, or painful parts of you as radiating light, gold, and beauty. Kintsugi teaches you that your broken places make you stronger and better than ever before. When you think you are broken, you can pick up the pieces, put them back together, and learn to embrace the cracks.

Many of us are struggling to be better, to recharge, or to keep up. We're constantly searching for the secret to self-improvement. But we know, on some deep level, that there is no secret. In order to heal and feel whole, we have to do the work.

For many years, I went through life with parts of my heart broken. I wasn't aware of it then, but I wasn't taking proper care of myself. I constantly felt as if I needed to keep going. I was very hard on myself. Inside, I carried a lot of lingering anger, sometimes sadness, and, almost always, a feeling of needing to belong. I never, ever felt quite "good enough," and was always seeking validation from outside.

When we were growing up, Mom and Dad were extremely tough on my older sister Jenni and me. They expected the very best from us, always. I would later come to realize that their philosophy was rooted in the traditional Japanese practices of *kaizen* (continuous improvement), *ganbatte* (do your best), *ki o tsukete* (take great care), and *kansha* (gratitude). Jenni and I were shown these practices at an early age, and we always carried them with us. When challenges inevitably arose, we used them as opportunities to heal, to work harder, to do better, to improve, and, ultimately, to be resilient through tough times.

The Japanese have a saying: *Oyano se wo mite ko wa sodatsu.*

"親の背を 見て、 子は 育つ。おやの せを みて、こは そだつ."

It means "Children learn by watching what their parents do, not by hearing what they say." My parents did not tell us about these Japanese practices. Instead, they showed us, always leading by example. They taught Jenni and me that if we followed these teachings, they would help us to become exactly who we are, and to find what we are looking for.

These practices will do the same for you. But the path I'm talking about is not the path of least resistance. It is more like a pavement that is slowly being laid before us as we take the next steps on our journey. Your journey is your story, unlike anyone else's. What makes you so special is the path that you are in the process of forging right now. Your story contains everything that makes you individually precious, and your story is a gift to the world.

On the surface, it may seem as if I am confident, and perhaps even strong. But the truth is, I am still working to fill my cracks. Across my heart you will find cracks caused by heartbreak, not feeling accepted by society, feeling "different," and childhood memories of never feeling good enough. For many years, living with these cracks made me feel incomplete.

For the first twelve years of my career, I never took a break. In perfect Japanese form, I worked hard and gave only my very best (known as *ganbatte,* which you'll learn more about on page 221). But I wasn't taking good care of myself. I never took breaks, other than the times when I would travel to see family during the holidays, and even then I never stopped working. I was afraid that if I stopped, others would catch up to me.

Then I began to study my heritage and piece together my past. It took a lot of hard work, but slowly, the cracks began to mend . . .

I have been traveling to Japan since I was in kindergarten. In recent years, Mom and I would meet up in Japan to visit family. Each time, she would note, "Don't forget to take a few of Baachan's (my Japanese grandmother's) things." Inevitably, after a few trips around the globe, some of the items broke. But I never threw them away. I worked on saving the pieces, so I could seal them with lacquer and dust them with gold.

I began painting on quiet weekends, sealing all the cracks with golden repair. The teacups you see on page 2 are my grandmother's, which have been repaired by kintsugi. This was a therapeutic practice for me, and a way to connect with an art form that has become reflective of my life.

In Japan, we honor our elders and treasure those who have passed. During the writing of this book, my sweet and loving Baachan passed away peacefully at age ninety-six. It was time to pay homage to the matriarch in our family, who raised four daughters just after World War II ended. Baachan

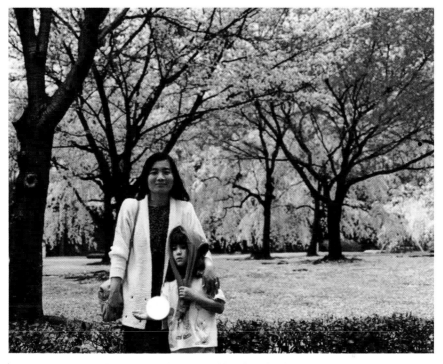

Kyoto, Japan, 1987: Mom and I: our endless love for *hanami*
(cherry blossom viewing) will live on.

was absolutely radiant, warm, and loving, and could always light up a room.

Mom, Jenni, and I went back to Japan for Baachan's one-year memorial
service. We wanted to pay our respects and honor her life, along with the
rest of our family. We planned to see the cherry blossoms together, for the
first time in over a decade.

During that trip, I went to study the traditional art of kintsugi with a
kintsugi master, Tsuyoshi Sensei. He generously allowed me to visit his
home art studio in Kyoto where he shared his work and taught me the
history of kintsugi.

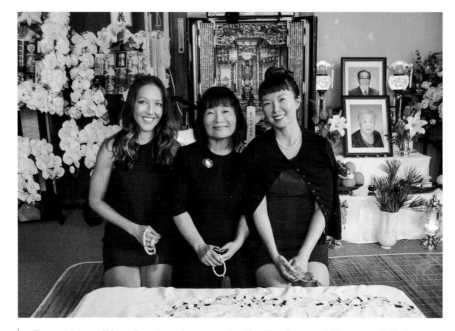

Beppu, Japan: Mom, Jenni, and me, praying for Baachan and Jiichan and their spirits.

I learned that kintsugi is a centuries-old art form that first became popular in the mid-fifteenth century. During the Muromachi period (1334–1573 AD), if a Japanese servant broke an object of their master's, they would turn the broken object over to a kintsugi artist to have it repaired. But it didn't stop there. In some cases, the servant would then take his or her own life as a sign of honesty and honor. (I know. It's super-extreme, and I couldn't believe it either.)

Luckily, this custom is no longer practiced. But over time, kintsugi became a national art form, and a way not just to mend broken vessels but also to celebrate imperfection. As I studied kintsugi with Tsuyoshi Sensei, I started to wonder how I could begin to repair the broken pieces in my own life.

One day soon after I'd returned home from this trip, I received a message from someone named Sarah, a perfect stranger. She invited me on a trip to Hana, Maui, for an experience called "the immersion." The itinerary was vague—I had no idea who else would be there, or what we'd be doing. I almost politely passed on the opportunity, but something inside urged me to accept.

I packed up my bags and flew nearly 5,000 miles to the magical island of Maui. When I landed, I was greeted by the staff for "the immersion" and began to meet the other guests. The first person I met was Paul, an amazing photographer from Chicago, followed by McKel, a nutritionist from Nashville. One by one, the Sprinter van at the Maui airport began to fill up with some of the most amazing people. The van took us on a three-hour excursion to Hana, a magical spot known for its healing, serenity, and peace.

There were fifty guests in all, and over the course of three days, we were encouraged to work on self-improvement through group workshops. The only thing considered mandatory was to simply be present.

By the third day, we had all learned so much about one another. We had shared deep-rooted pain, illness, personal struggles, deep loss, and deaths in our families—everything. Midway through our class that day, our instructor asked if anything had come up for us. Everyone fell silent. The truth was, a lot had come up for me. Though I hadn't felt comfortable sharing my story, a tiny little voice inside me said, "Go, Candice, it's your turn. It's okay." I took a deep breath, and slowly walked to the front of the class. Forty-nine pairs of eyes were all on me. I started to tremble and my palms were super-clammy, but I opened my mouth to speak.

"Hi guys, I'm Candice. I'm from New York City by way of San Diego,"

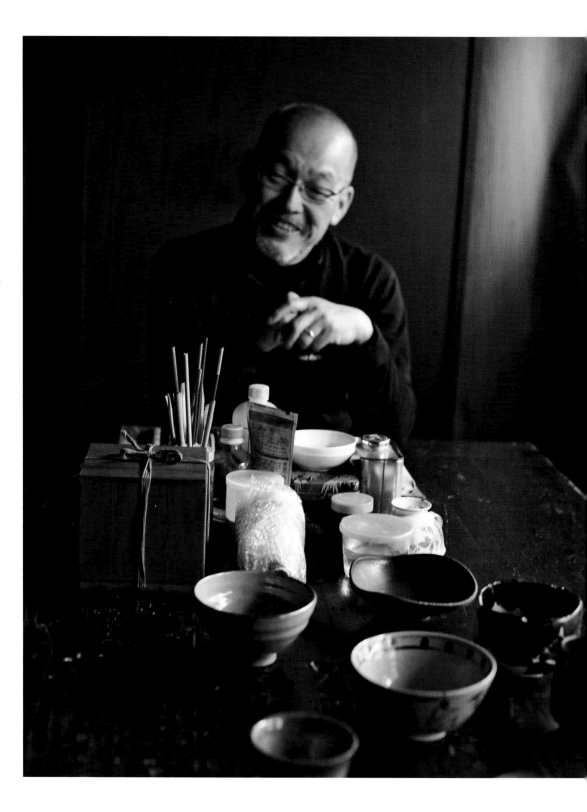

I started. "About a year ago, my best friend left me." I went on to explain how one day, my boyfriend of a few years came home to the apartment we shared and suddenly told me he was leaving. Thirty minutes later, he was on his way to the airport. And just like that, the life I had was broken open.

As I shared my story, the group at the immersion was so silent, you could hear a pin drop. I told them how I had tried to soldier on through the pain. I shared how my family encouraged me not to ruminate, but to move on immediately. In traditional Japanese form, I had been raised to believe there was no time to feel sorry for myself.

As I looked around the room with teary eyes, I saw tears begin to roll down others' cheeks. I'll never forget what it was like to look around a room of forty-nine faces—professional athletes, producers, writers, directors, singers, actors, you name it—and feel that they understood how it felt to be broken.

Our instructor then told me to place two hands over my heart. The people near me were told to put their hands on me, and the rest of the group was to attach themselves to someone who was touching me. Forty-nine minds and one hundred hands were all linking back to my heart. Then our teacher encouraged everyone to send me compassion. A flood of love and energy washed over me. I can still feel the power of that energy to this day. I understood that each and every piece of me could be put back together. I also understood that I wasn't alone.

In this safe space, our masks came off, and everyone began to share their

Kyoto, Japan: Tsuyoshi Sensei shares with us the history of kintsugi.

own cracks. This experience showed me how *everyone* has places where they are broken. Everyone has the power to heal themselves, and to come out even stronger.

Over the course of our time together, a group of perfect strangers turned into a support group. We shared our stories and our secrets. It was so comforting to see that all these people, whom I considered to be strong, successful leaders, were imperfect. And their imperfections made them even more extraordinary.

Each of the stories shared that day gave others permission to share and repair. The more we talked, the more we all accepted that it's okay to show your cracks. While we may not always want to be brave, we must remember that when we put up walls or don't share our story, we do a disservice to everyone around us.

Through kintsugi, we learn it is okay to hurt and grieve. It is okay to be vulnerable. It is okay to accept and allow yourself the time to share, to open up, to exercise compassion. After the immersion, I felt more mindful and aware. I was more attentive to the present moment and able to experience joy in the little things. But I was going to have to learn how to mend my cracks on my own, in real life. I was going to have to do the work. Once I got back home to New York, the practice became more real to me. I was going to have to do the work of golden repair on my own. Yet I held on to the sunshine, the gratitude, the acceptance, and the growth from my experience with a group of strangers.

Wherever you are right now, I urge you to take a solid look back on all that you have experienced, and all that you have healed and sealed from. More often than not, we do not pay attention and we do not track our progress. We live in a culture where we expect perfection and condemn ourselves when we are not perfect or when things don't go our way. But sometimes, it takes years of persistence, hard work, and dedication to better hone and own your perfected craft before you can see the bigger picture.

You already have many cracks that have been honored and sealed. Have a think on that, and give yourself credit for going through this journey of life. It's a pretty amazing feeling when you finally realize you are right where you're meant to be.

kintsugi marks your progress, so you do not forget.

Like a map of your heart, kintsugi shows us the lessons and reveals the truth. As much as the struggle, the pain, the trials and tribulations sucked, even when things were *not* your fault, all of life's hurt can be mended through golden repair. When we change our mind-set about our past, we have come out of the struggles as a much more beautiful and refined version of ourselves. Your kintsugi cracks become gold by doing the work.

kintsugi teaches you to be kind to yourself.

The spirit of kintsugi is also about forgiveness. It's a practice of self-love. Accepting your cracks means being accepting and loving toward yourself. You must forgive yourself first, before you are capable of forgiving another. As you work toward this, you'll see that the most beautiful, meaningful parts of yourself are the ones that have been broken, mended, and healed.

kintsugi is a continuous practice.

Learning is the key to kintsugi, and we never stop learning. I have consistently spoken these soft words to my tough heart, "Candice, you have much to learn." To practice Japanese wellness, you must approach it with an open and honest heart. I am committed to these practices, and committed to continuously improving every day. But I promise you, all it takes is openness, and you can learn.

your cracks make you beautiful.

The physical art of kintsugi is beautiful, but that's not what this book is about. The part I find moving, and what I want to share with you, is the analogy of embracing your past wounds, scars, pain, and internal struggle, and accepting their value. Your deepest pain, your biggest fears—all the struggles you've gone through—have forever changed you. If you could see my heart, you would see there are golden cracks all over it. Some run deep, some are still being sealed, and many more are still to come. Your heart looks very much the same. Kintsugi is life's way of saying, "nobody's perfect." The path is not straight. In fact, your hardest challenges, deepest wounds, and greatest fears are actually among the most beautiful, precious, and admirable parts of you.

you will have to do the work.

What is "the work," you ask? I've broken it down into ten principles:

Wabi-sabi—Admire imperfection

Gaman—Live with great resilience

Eiyōshoku—Nourish your body

Ki o tsukete—Learn to take care

Ganbatte—Always do your best

Kaizen—Continuously improve

Shikata ga nai—Accept what cannot be helped

Yuimaru—Care for your inner circle

Kansha—Cultivate sincere gratitude

Osettai—Be of service to others, welcoming gifts

Along with kintsugi, these are the practices that have helped me. It's almost a step-by-step program. These are the ten philosophies that guide my work ethic, my inspiration, and my authenticity, and they keep me going.

We'll delve into each one, along with my daily practices, in the coming chapters.

Hajimemashō. はじめましょう。始めましょう. Let's begin.

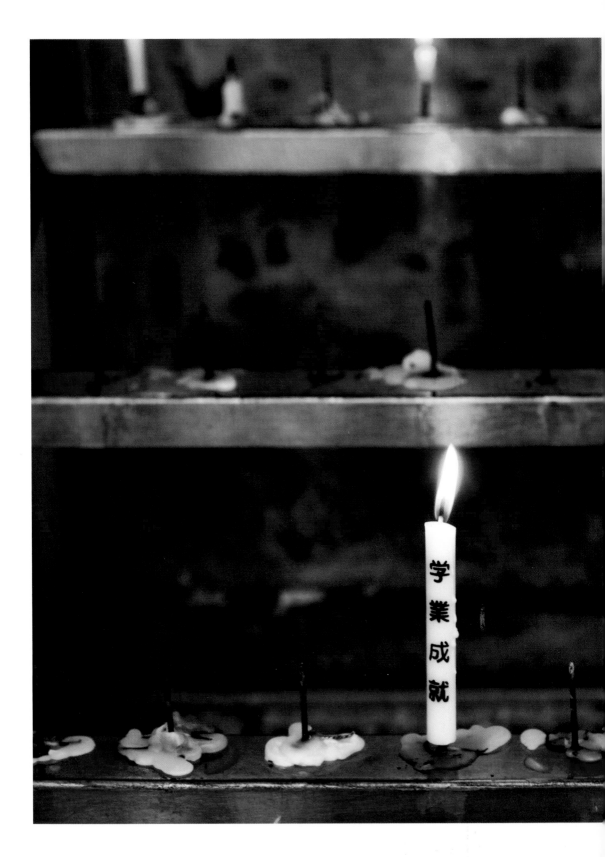

2

wabi-sabi

侘び寂び, わびさび

celebrate

imperfection

| Shikoku Island temple, where millions come to visit, pray, and find peace.

MY MOTHER ALWAYS SAYS, "LIFE CANNOT BE PERFECT FOREVER."

When I was growing up, I used to think it was a sad thing to say, but as I've gotten older I've come to appreciate her perspective. She says these words matter-of-factly, because they are true. Life can't be perfect forever. In other words, life will exhaust you, it will crush you sometimes—and that's okay. Holding ourselves up to a "perfect" standard is ultimately defeating, because perfection is fleeting. And imperfection is nothing to be afraid of.

My mom's attitude toward imperfection is rooted in the Japanese idea of *wabi-sabi*. Like kintsugi, wabi-sabi celebrates life's imperfections, its tough stretches, and even its dark corners. It reminds us that life is transient, imperfection is natural, and there is beauty to be found in simplicity.

Wabi-sabi: The word *wabi* refers to being alone, or loneliness (*wabi shi* means "alone") In poetry, the word *wabi* typically refers to something that is simple, humble, and in line with nature. It can also mean a simple, austere beauty. (Think of a monk, who is at peace living with very little.) Meanwhile, *sabi* refers to the passage of time, the process of aging, and the fleeting nature of all things.

You might be familiar with wabi-sabi as an aesthetic or design idea. In Japan, our architecture, pottery, and home décor is often simple but elegant. A wabi-sabi approach to design embraces simplicity and imperfection. For example, a vase of wilting flowers may be just as beautiful and appreciated as a vase of freshly picked blossoms. Similarly, wabi-sabi might celebrate an architectural flaw, like the crumbling façade of an old building. In the Western world, where we are often obsessed with symmetry and perfection, wabi-sabi can help us appreciate and reframe what we think of as "ugly."

The concept of wabi-sabi dates back to the twelfth century. Japan had gone through a brutal civil war, and the imperial court culture shifted to a military regime ruled by shoguns. For much of the population, it felt like death was always around the corner. Within this changing landscape, the concept of wabi-sabi emerged to capture the beauty that is found in transience and impermanence.

The aesthetic side of wabi-sabi came about in the fifteenth and sixteenth centuries, through the emergence of the Japanese tea ceremony. These aristocratic gatherings became simpler and sparer, and began to take on the aesthetic that is now widely associated with Japan—simple earth-toned pottery, cracked or asymmetrical teacups, and iron teapots. To this day, the Japanese tea ceremony is known for its beauty and elegance.

In modern times, we can see why the Japanese would embrace this philosophy. After all, the land of Japan is far from perfect, the weather can be extreme (with cold winters, hot summers, and rainy seasons), and there's always the chance of a natural disaster, like an earthquake or tsunami. But instead of living in fear (or feeling like they've gotten a bad deal), the Japanese accept that there's always a bit of uncertainty and darkness to be found in the big picture of life. Perfection seems wonderful, but it is always fleeting. Good times cannot and will not exist forever, and the more you embrace and plan for the fact that tough times will happen, the easier it is to survive them.

When I was last in Japan, I had the honor of spending time at the temples in Kōyasan and in Shikoku with Buddhist monks. To say that monks embrace imperfection, simplicity, and transience is an understatement. The monks shave their heads, turning away from vanity, as it is an unnecessary distraction. And yet, these men and women radiate the most beautiful light in the world. They devote their lives to prayer, sending light into dark places. In order to do that, they first must understand and accept that dark places exist. The monks know better than anyone that there is beauty to be found in distortion, in wilted flowers, in a broken heart, in our missteps and mistakes. There is beauty in struggle.

Accepting imperfection has been a lifelong challenge for me. It started when I was a young child. Growing up in a predominantly white neighborhood as the daughter of a Japanese immigrant mother and Polish immigrant father, I felt *different*. I was brought up differently than the other kids—my parents were strict and wouldn't tolerate anything less than my best—and, obviously, I looked different.

As I got older, I was teased for being different. Kids asked mean questions and sometimes called me racist names. Like any young girl, I wanted to be beautiful, popular, and accepted. I wanted people to like me for who I was.

When I was fifteen, a modeling agency approached me at my school's "career day." They told me I was tall, lanky, and "exotic." It was certainly unexpected, but I was curious and decided to give it a try. From there, modeling became a side gig that grew into something more. All throughout college I continued to work as a fit model (meaning a live mannequin for fashion designers, not to be confused with a "fitness" model) and print model. I worked all over the U.S. and the globe in the name of fashion.

While the lifestyle was glam, always chasing perfection was not. I had designers measuring my thighs, butt, waist, and hips. I body-shamed my-

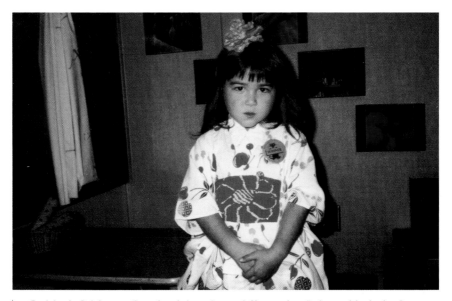

| Carlsbad, California: Preschool days. I was different, but I always liked who I was.

self constantly, and my deep-rooted love for cooking called just as my modeling career peaked. I had to learn to balance culinary school with tiny bikinis and sample-size jeans. (How fun!) For a decade, I told myself I had to be perfect. At our weekly measurements, if you were a quarter-inch off perfection, you could lose your job.

Although I no longer get measured on a regular basis, those days of chasing perfection are still ingrained in my mind. As I've gotten older, I'm not really concerned with the circumference of my hips, but the feeling of needing to be perfect still haunts me. I constantly have to remind myself that not only is perfection a myth, but that imperfection is nothing to fear.

Just as wabi-sabi can teach us to appreciate the beauty of a wilted flower or a chipped teacup, it can also teach us to appreciate—and reconsider—

our physical forms. Whether it's a scar, laugh lines, freckles, or gray hairs, wabi-sabi recognizes that difference is beauty.

Imperfection is the natural condition of everything. So much of beauty is in the eye of the beholder, and the more we open ourselves up to wabi-sabi, the more we begin to appreciate how our differences are what make us beautiful. You know how a leather jacket, Converse high tops, or jeans just look cooler when they're slightly worn in? That's wabi-sabi.

I now find beauty in unexpected places. I find it in wrinkles. I find it in the way the sunlight hits the branches of a bare tree in the winter. I find beauty in kind eyes and kind hearts. I find beauty in the most giving people. I find beauty in humble people, and those who are honest and sincere.

Here are a few more things you can do to help bring wabi-sabi into your perspective:

reset your way of thinking: The changing of seasons is a nice prompt to get back to nature. You can go for a simple walk, hike, or run, and take the time to contemplate. Observe the imperfections all around you. Whether it's the changing colors of the leaves, the moss growing on the rocks, or moldy bark on a tree, it's all in the eye of the beholder. Imperfection is part of the natural order.

trade judgment for acceptance: We all have preconceived ideas about the people we meet—and we are quick to judge one another. Everyone has an inner beauty, and if you choose not to look through a lens of judgment, you will be astounded by the beauty you see.

forgive: People aren't perfect. They make mistakes, or, as my friend Richard once told me, "people will malfunction." Part of a wabi-sabi practice is learning to accept and forgive. It isn't always easy, but it is better to let go and forgive than to live with a knot in your stomach or a grudge in your heart. You'll be able to sleep easier at night, and you'll make room in your life for more positive experiences.

stop comparing: It's all too easy in the age of social media to compare ourselves to others. But if we stop comparing, we can allow ourselves to find more peace and acceptance. Each morning, before I touch any of my electronic devices, I like to meditate. It gives me a chance to clear my head and erase any judgment, anxiety, worry, or doubt that I have about my life or my future.

simplify: Balance is about slowing down and appreciating what we have. Practicing wabi-sabi can also mean simplifying your life. You already have everything you need right at this very moment. None of the bells and whistles can come with you when you leave. And hey, guess what? Shiny new things won't solve anything, and they aren't important.

work on self-acceptance: This is probably one of the hardest things we can learn. Self-acceptance is a process, but I've found it helpful to spend time alone. When you're alone you don't have to worry about a persona. You can take off your mask, and just do you. Accept that every person is flawed, including you. Believe that everyone is doing their best with what they have to work with. That includes you. Let up on yourself and remember that there is no standard you need to measure up to. You're really special the way that you are. (It's not just your mom telling you this, it's me!) Your imperfections make you unique.

look at wisdom as beauty: My sister and I often have conversations about how wonderful it would be if society valued character and integrity as much as it did beauty and power. Appreciate someone who has taught you something, or inspired you, or whose presence has brought you enjoyment. If there are elders in your life who are close to you, whether it's a grandparent, a neighbor, or a mentor, spend time with them, and appreciate their wisdom.

I was once told, "You can't pour from an empty cup." When I finally let go of my need for a perfect relationship, I realized I didn't need anyone else to make me great. Then something crazy happened. I began to accept the imperfect moments, the imperfect people, the imperfect days, my imperfect self. I began to accept the difficult conversations, the struggle, the compromise, the discomfort.

So much of wabi-sabi is about changing your mind-set to see life from a different perspective. Appreciate the struggles just a bit more, and life will feel a little bit easier. Without the struggles, you will never be able to tap into your strength and your real potential. Sometimes, the goal of living isn't all about winning. Sometimes it's about being, enduring, experiencing, learning, trying, failing. When you come out on the other side, you'll be grateful for the beautiful, imperfect view.

mono no aware

物の哀れ, もののあわれ

the pathos of life, a gentle sadness

As a culture, Americans are somewhat obsessed with positivity. From a young age, we are taught to approach life with a positive, can-do attitude. American children are taught to look on the bright side, and that if they think good thoughts, they will manifest good things.

Japanese culture embraces a more realistic approach. Life can't always be perfect. There will be challenges, and if you expect them, they won't take you by surprise. In Japanese culture, we are taught to embrace the difficulties with empathy and mindfulness.

The phrase *mono no aware* literally translates to "the pathos of things." Like wabi-sabi, it refers to the transience of life. There is a mild sadness in this idea—mourning or grieving the fleeting nature of life—and in Japanese culture this is accepted as a reality rather than something to fight.

Mono no aware is about seeing things as they are. Sometimes they will be good, and sometimes they will be bad. Without darkness, light cannot exist. *Mono no aware* teaches us that while bad things do inevitably happen, it is our chance to practice empathy and compassion for others.

I have an eighty-two-year-old sensei friend, Yamazaki-san, who lives in the Noto Peninsula of Japan. Yamazaki is a former college professor and a beloved mentor to me. He and I write letters to each other, and I always find a light and wisdom in his correspondence that is hard to describe. He recently wrote me a note that sums up the idea of *mono no aware* beautifully:

能登の海の夕景きれいです。

「黄金の波穂の奥に日が沈む　縄文海人ら銛 (もり) を研ぎけむ」

Pious people worship the rising sun, waiting for the sun to rise out of the sea or to set. A beautiful and moving sight! In my fishing village in Noto, we can also enjoy the sun setting into the sea.

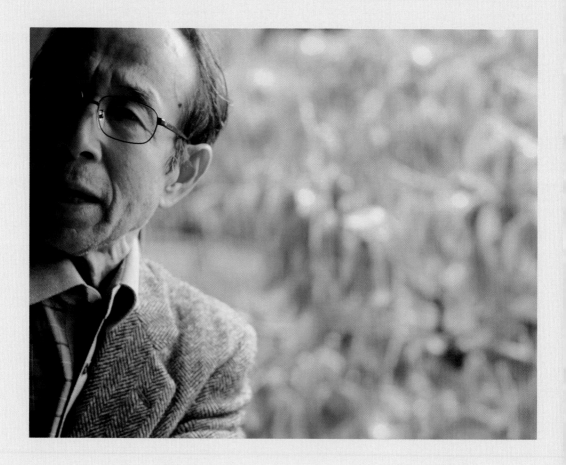

Most Japanese people know "The Crane Wife," which is a story of a bewitched bird that married a poor but kindhearted man. When it was retold by Mr. Junji Kinoshita in 1949, it leapt to fame. His version is called "Yūzuru," the literal meaning of which is "Twilight Crane." The last scene is: "In time the crane wife was seen to fly up and away in the twilight sky." Beautiful, but sorrowful.

Since I came across the folk tale I have enjoyed seeing the sun set, especially watching fishermen row out to sea for night fishing, their boats moving in a dim silhouette against the glow of the western sky.

When we embrace the concept of *mono no aware*, we accept that in every life, some bad will come. It is okay to be sad, it is healthy to feel deeply, and it is completely normal to struggle. Allow yourself to feel the full range of your emotions, both positive *and* negative. These are the moments during which we can better learn to dive deep and accept ourselves through each facet of life. Our lives are forever changing, as are we.

Noto Peninsula, Japan: Yamazaki-san, my eighty-two-year-old mentor and sensei.

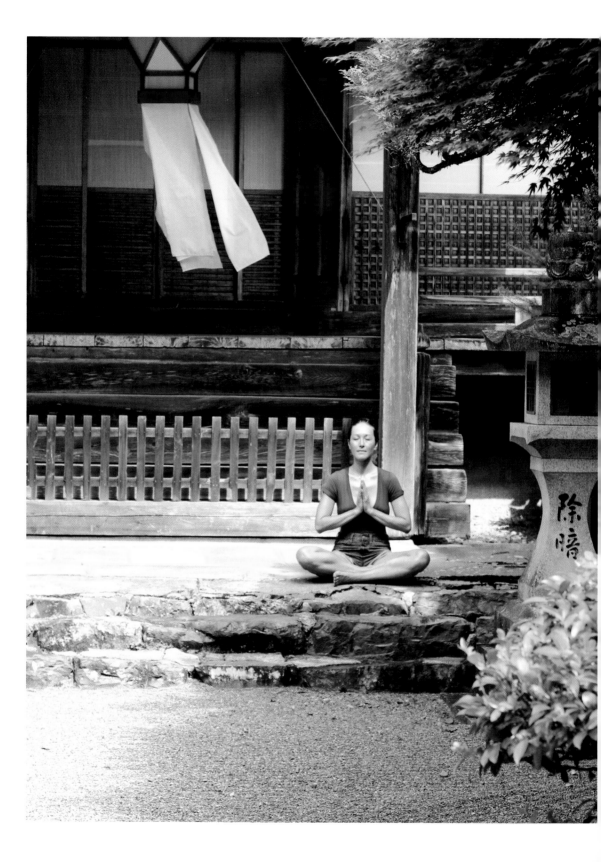

g a m a n

我慢, がまん

endure pain

with patience,

resilience, and

tolerance

IN 2011, JAPAN WAS HIT BY A DEVASTATING SERIES OF EVENTS. A 9.1-magnitude earthquake—the largest earthquake ever to hit Japan—took place 231 miles northeast of Tokyo. The quake caused a massive tsunami with 30-foot waves, damaging several nuclear reactors at the Fukushima Daiichi power plant. The disaster claimed over 22,000 lives and cost billions of dollars in damage.

As the rest of the world grieved the enormous loss and sent humanitarian aid, the Japanese people did what they always do.

They endured.

Beginning at an early age, the Japanese teach their children the principle of *gaman*—the ability to endure by remaining calm, patient, and resilient. When a Japanese child is hungry or complaining, her mom will respond to her, *"Gaman!"* Traditionally, the Japanese do not complain or react dramatically to challenging times. Rather, they prefer to be still and allow the storm to pass, as they quietly endure the changes along the course.

We need not wait for a storm to enter the picture in order to practice gaman. We can practice gaman in our everyday lives. No matter what is going on around you—a stressful workday, a bad mood (we've all been there), a misunderstanding—you can learn to practice resilience.

For me, gaman typically takes the form of my self-care routine. Meditating each morning helps to ease my mind, while getting some form of daily exercise helps me to stay calm and focused. Getting the right nutrition (more on that in the next chapter) and a good night's sleep gives me the strength to endure the challenges each day brings.

Gaman will take practice and work. As a New Yorker, stress and struggle are part of my everyday life—and truth be told, we tend to focus on the struggle. Whenever I think of reacting to a difficult situation, I take a deep breath and try to remember the Japanese phrase *shō ga nai,* meaning "it cannot be helped." We all experience struggles and setbacks, and we all feel pain. It is to our greatest advantage to work together, to be patient, and to cultivate more peace.

Gaman also teaches us not to make a situation worse by elevating the drama. Stop, take a moment, and remember to breathe. Once you've had a chance to pause and assess things calmly—only then—take action. As my mom says, "Gaman is about being tolerant, holding back your desires or anger, and ultimately letting them go. Don't let these negative thoughts or urges take over your life. If you keep holding on to grudges in your mind, this creates stress. Practicing gaman reduces stress."

But how do you actually practice gaman? What if you are currently going through a particularly hard time? How do you stay resilient? I have experienced—and have seen so many of my friends through—situations where it seemed as if things would never get better. Every time, it seemed hopeless. Every time, we not only healed but came out stronger on the other side.

If you're going through some sort of setback, whether it's heartbreak, a job change, or the loss of a loved one, remember we each grieve in different ways. Acknowledge the fact that your process will be your own. Allow yourself the room to move through the stages of grief, and take good care of yourself. Eat nourishing foods, go on long walks, and spend time with people who care about you and have your best interests at heart. Let your family and friends serve as a sounding board. When I was going through a difficult time recently, I also found it was helpful to avoid alcohol until I could see clearly again.

No matter what, let yourself rest. Sometimes when you're going through a tough time, all you want to do is sleep, and that's okay. Sleep as much as you can. It will help you to recharge. Listen to your body more than you normally would. It will let you know what you need.

Rest assured that time is going to be life's greatest healer. Life has a process, and you can trust in it.

In the meantime, there are things you can do to condition yourself and prepare for the storm.

take action: As my mother taught by example, if you don't like something, don't complain. Instead, take action to change it. Instead of feeling sorry for yourself, or ruminating on a bad situation, create change. Then get out there and focus on doing more of what feels good and will help you in the long run.

eat fresh: Do your best to eat fresh foods at every meal. Food is information to the cells in your body. When you nourish your body with living foods, you will feel more alive.

cut back: A few years ago, I cut excess sugar out of my diet and swapped coffee for matcha, and it has done wonders for my life. I feel less jittery and anxious; my mind feels clear, and I am more able to focus on the tasks at hand. I don't feel groggy when I wake up in the mornings, and all day long I feel more energized. Cutting back on the things you consume on a regular basis can be a great way to gauge what feels good versus what doesn't.

get moving: The Japanese (especially the people of Okinawa) have some of the longest life spans in the world. One of the secrets of their longevity is their dedication to incorporating movement into their everyday lives. I encourage you to move your body each and every day. Regular exercise has really helped to clear my head of anxiety and depression. I like to alternate different types of movement to keep my muscles guessing and to keep my mind from getting bored.

socialize, in real life: Connection is what keeps us together. Socializing with others helps to grow your own self-love and self-care. And I don't just mean the group text on your phone. Being part of a social circle—and finding time to invest in that circle and community—helps improve your quality of life and boosts longevity. Keeping in touch with friends from different stages and parts of your life—whether it's a weekly phone call, annual visit, or a vacation taken together to an exotic locale—can seem like a big-time commitment, but I promise it's one that pays huge dividends. Some of my closest friendships have endured decades of separation and we remain as tight as ever after. When someone knows you for that amount of time, they've been there through thick and thin. Treasure and prize your true friendships in real life.

group workouts: To that end, I'm in love with combining movement and socialization. Group fitness is what gets me up and out of the house in the morning. There are so many classes out there, and you can surely find something that appeals to you. Try a group run, boot camp workout, cycling class, barre class, yoga class, or even just a community class (like cooking or gardening) that gets you out of your routine and connecting more, in real life.

group meditation: Group meditation classes (and even group meditation centers) are becoming increasingly common. Meditating with others provides a quiet, supportive environment, and guided meditations are great for beginners. Making the time to sit and look inward really helps to focus your mind and energy.

make peace: A huge part of adapting to the lives we are given is letting go of expectations—both those we set for ourselves and those others have of us. There are many things we can't control, whether financial stress, a job loss, emotional turmoil, or the actions of a boss or a friend. The sooner we learn that we cannot control everything and make an effort to let go of those things we cannot change, the more we are able to find peace.

stay the course: The principles of gaman—staying the course no matter what—can also be used in a practical way to push yourself to new levels of endurance and achievement. Stay focused on the journey, and have faith that you are headed exactly where you're meant to be. I personally like to use the mind-set of gaman during a challenging moment, or to push myself to do difficult things. You might use gaman to help you study harder, to work better, or to accomplish more in your day. If you use the art of gaman to endure, you can get through anything. See nothing as an obstacle but rather as a challenge, and think about how good you are going to feel once you get through the fight!

Sometimes practicing gaman is simply about letting go and being still. The greatest lesson I have learned is to let go of what was not meant to be. Whether it's a relationship, a job, or a hoped-for adventure, there is power in gracefully letting something go. There is power in knowing that wherever you are in this moment is right where you are meant to be. Even if you are deep in the trenches, you are resilient. Even when all you feel like doing is crying, you are a ray of light.

When you begin to let go, you open up your heart to wonderful new people and exciting new opportunities. Don't let anyone or anything dim your light. Remember the practice of gaman, and shine on with resilience and grace.

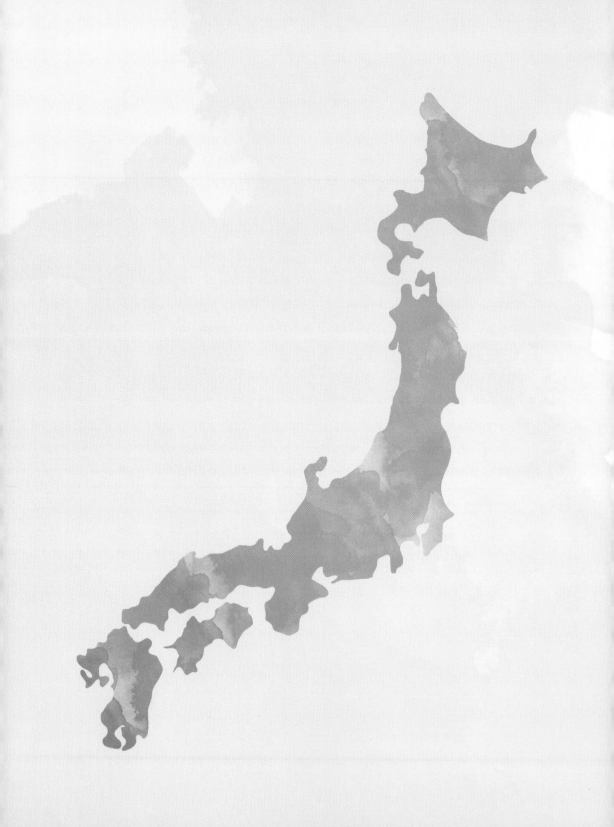

II

nourish

eiyōshoku

栄養食, えいようしょく

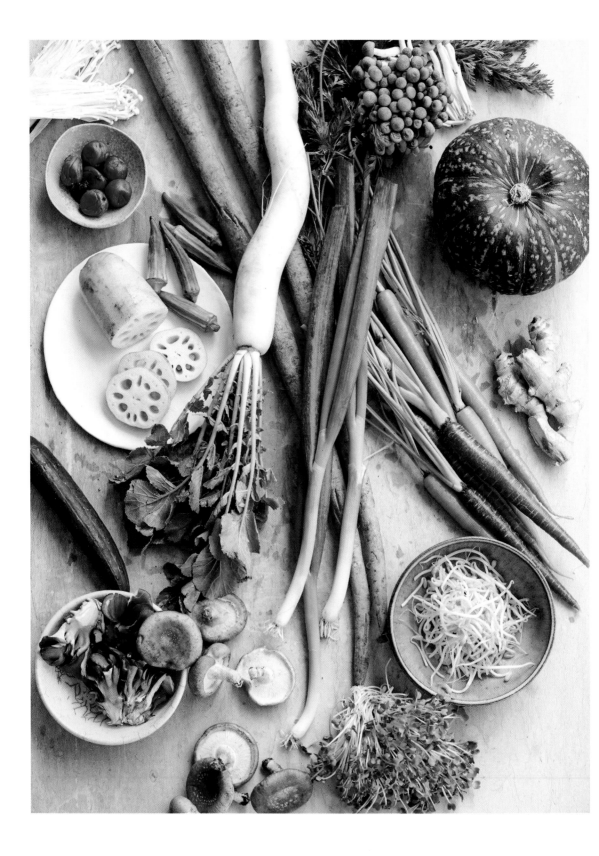

4

ryōri

料理, りょうり

cooking

Cooking and eating nourishing foods are the foundations of my kintsugi-inspired self-care. The act of nourishing our bodies is a simple thing, but its effects are profound. Eating well allows us to respect and honor our body's needs.

When I say to eat nutritiously, I don't mean that you have to eat less. I always tell my friends who are dieting to *stop* what they're doing and listen to their bodies instead! No body wants deprivation or restriction. Every body needs nutrients from real, whole foods to flourish—the same foods that nourished my ancestors and your ancestors for centuries. That means lots of fresh produce, healthy protein, fermented foods, and unprocessed grains. Simple, seasonal, delicious food. Remember, Baachan lived until she was ninety-six (and her skin glowed all her life!). If we want to learn the secrets of Japanese wellness, we'd be wise to emulate the lifestyle of my elders!

And the best way to nourish yourself is to cook for yourself. Cooking is the only art form that utilizes all five senses—I almost see it as a form of meditation. Even when I'm not in the mood to cook, even when I don't feel like going to the grocery store or taking one single pot out of the cabinet, I always find that I get into a comfortable, familiar rhythm once I start cooking. And after I've made a meal with my own hands, I'm tremendously grateful for the food that will nourish me in mind and body. Best of all, food just tastes better when you cook it yourself.

Cooking comes from the heart; it is a language of love we must continue to speak to one another.

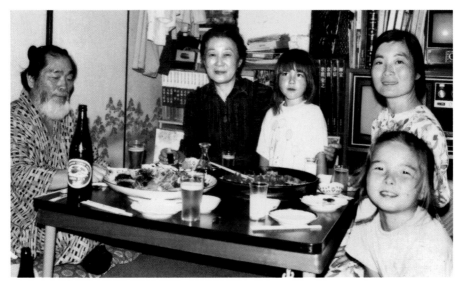

Beppu, Japan, 1987: Me and my Jiichan and Baachan. Growing up, we rarely missed a meal together. This was the power of *issho*, something that we should not lose sight of. It is a practice we should all commit to: more meals together as a family.

east meets west in the kitchen

I started helping my mom in the kitchen when I was about four years old. I can remember looking up at her with her long, dark, beautiful hair, her eye for perfection, her palate for taste, and her hard-working hands. I could barely see over the counter, but I can remember everything: the smell, the sound, the feeling, the passion, the taste! My mother was talented, she was good at everything, but to me, she shined most in the kitchen. I am forever grateful for the magic she has passed on to me, with my wide-*hapa* eyes looking over at her for decades. I was happiest when I was in the kitchen with her.

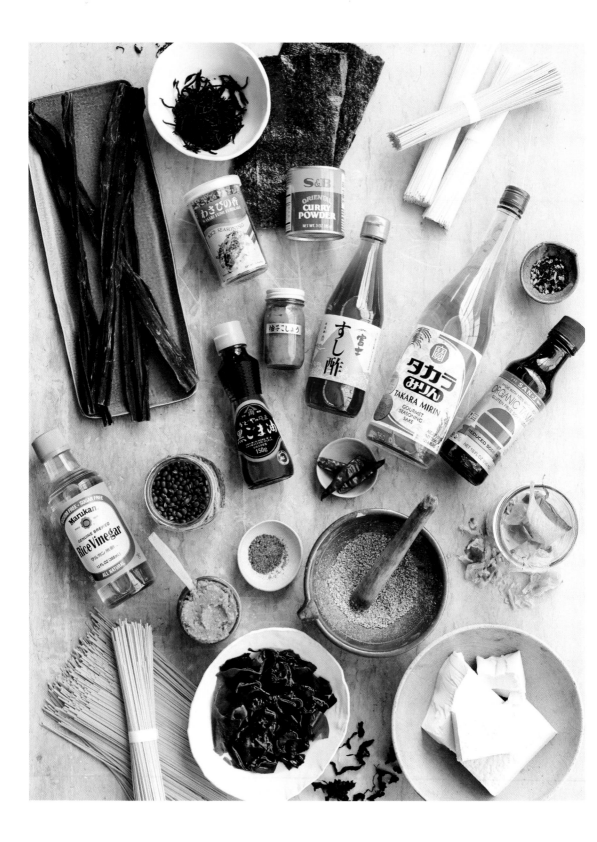

Mom and I made everything together, from homemade sushi to *sekihan* (red bean rice), mountain-rice mix to *miso shiru* (soup), *tsukemono* (Japanese pickles), *okonomiyaki*, *soba*, *sōmen* (cold noodles), *gyōza*, *udon*, and, of course, *mochi*.

In this book, I've included a selection of recipes that utilize Eastern and Western methods, techniques, and ingredients. Please note that these are not all super-traditional Japanese recipes, but instead represent an eclectic mix of my family's recipes and my Japanese-Californian heritage. I like to think that my mom perfected this hybrid cuisine, and her inspired dishes made an imprint on my soul. I may have gone to culinary school and cooked in restaurants, but Mom taught me how to *really* cook.

japanese pantry basics

You don't have to overhaul your pantry to make the recipes in this book, but it is helpful to stock up on a few specialty items before you begin cooking. You can order all these ingredients online or find them at your local Japanese grocer.

kanbutsu
乾物, かんぶつ
dry pantry items

seaweed

kombu (japanese kelp; 昆布, こんぶ): A Japanese seaweed that's frequently used to make *kombu dashi* (stock/soup), kombu is an anti-inflammatory food that's high in iron. Kombu may help keep your metabolism in check and is full of vitamins A, B_2, B_3, and B_6. Kombu can be cut or broken into small pieces and boiled to make kombu dashi. It's also used to add umami flavor to other dishes. Purchase kombu dried and store in an airtight container at room temperature for up to one year.

nori (japanese seaweed; 海苔, のり): Nori is the paper-like seaweed used to wrap sushi and hand rolls. Nori is made by growing, harvesting, straining, cutting, pressing, and drying seaweed. It is rich in minerals and is an amazing source of potassium, magnesium, calcium, iron, and vitamins A, B_{12}, C, and E. Nori may help to keep your skin glowing and your bones and teeth strong! Purchase it dried in square flat sheets and store in an airtight container at room temperature for up to three months. If your nori ever becomes soggy, you can lightly and *carefully* toast it quickly over an open flame (low heat) on a gas stovetop.

wakame (わかめ): A Japanese seaweed typically used in miso soup and reconstituted in water for salads, wakame is filled with vitamin B_{12}, iron, manganese, and brain-healthy omega-3 fatty acids. And like all seaweeds, it's a great source of iodine. Savor wakame in heart-warming recipes like my Red Potato + Onion Shiitake Miso Soup (page 103). Purchase it dried and reconstitute in water for cooking. Store dried wakame in an airtight container at room temperature for up to one year.

hijiki (ひじき): Hijiki is small, dark seaweed harvested from coastlines in Asia. Hijiki can be found in many popular seaweed salads and macrobiotic dishes. It is full of nutrients and minerals like iron, potassium, magnesium, calcium, fiber, and vitamin C. Purchase it dried and reconstitute it in water for about twenty minutes, making sure to strain and squeeze out excess liquid prior to using. You can store it reconstituted and drained in an airtight container in the fridge for up to a week. Store dried hijiki in an airtight container at room temperature for up to one year.

rice

gohan (cooked rice; 御飯 ご飯 ごはん): Gohan is the staple of Japanese cuisine. The Japanese consume so much rice that in Japan, the word *gohan* can also mean "dinner" or "meal." You will find a side of white rice at most meals, to be consumed with tsukemono (Japanese pickles), miso soup, or the main course. White rice contains protein, magnesium, phosphorus, manganese, selenium, iron, and folic acid. It's best to purchase Japanese rice at a Japanese market. Mom and I personally purchase Calrose rice that is grown and harvested in our home state of California. Store in an airtight container for up to one year.

genmai (brown rice; 玄米, げんまい): Brown rice contains the external germ attached to the rice grain, and is packed with nutrients like selenium, manganese, copper, and fiber. Eating more whole grains like brown rice can help you maintain a healthy weight, and may help reduce cholesterol.

mochigome (sweet mochi rice; 餅米, もちごめ): This is a glutinous, short-grain rice used to create *mochi (omochi)*, *senbei* (せんべい), *arare* (あられ), *sekihan* (page 125), sweet cakes, and tea cakes. Mochigome is a sweet, sticky, and chewy rice grain. Although it is a "glutinous" rice by description, it contains no gluten. You can find mochigome at the Japanese store, sometimes also labeled "sweet mochi rice" and "sticky rice." Store in a cool, dry, dark place, sealed well, for up to six months.

mochiko (sweet rice flour; もち粉, もちこ): This is a delicious milled rice flour used to make Japanese mochi and my Coconut Mochi Squares (page 197). Sweet rice flour is also known as "mochiko" and is gluten-free. Mochiko is used throughout this book to make recipes like mochi and *dango*.

sauces, vinegars, and oils

shōyu (soy sauce; 醤油, しょうゆ): Shōyu is a Japanese staple seasoning made of fermented soybeans. I've used shōyu in every one of my cookbooks—I can't cook without it! Nothing can compare to the depth, flavor, and umami of shōyu. I recommend that you use a low-sodium soy sauce, as most traditional varieties pack a heavy dose of salt.

goma abura (toasted sesame oil; ごま油, ごまあぶら): Rich in fragrance and flavor, dark in color, toasted sesame oil is one of my favorite oils to cook with, next to coconut! The deep flavor and essence of goma abura in Japanese cuisine has no comparison. You'll love this nutty and earthy toasted treat to top off your salads, in marinades, and in soups. I always stir-fry and sauté my Japanese dishes with *goma abura*!

kome su (rice vinegar; 米酢, こめす): I love the flavor of acidity in my foods. There's a brightness you can taste on your palate with vinegar.

all about soy sauce

shōyu (soy sauce; 醤油, しょうゆ)

Regular soy sauce, known as *koikuchi shōyu* in Japanese, is a staple seasoning made of fermented soybeans and wheat (about 50:50, but the ratio may vary) plus enzymes and salt. Shōyu is a staple ingredient in most Asian recipes and households. It contains vitamin K_2, protein, vitamin B_3, and manganese. Store, refrigerated, for up to one year.

tamari jōyu (tamari soy sauce; たまり醤油, たまりじょうゆ)

Tamari shōyu or jōyu is a delicious wheat-free seasoning and substitute for soy sauce. However, if you have a gluten intolerance, be sure to read labels carefully, as not *all* tamari is wheat-free. Like soy sauce, tamari is fermented, making it great for your gut health. I recommend looking for organic San-J brand tamari at your local health food store, major grocery store, or Japanese market. Store, refrigerated, for up to one year.

gen-en tamari jōyu (reduced-sodium soy sauce; 減塩たまり醤油, げんえんたまりじょうゆ)

Gen-en tamari jōyu is my most recommended shōyu in this book, especially if you are looking to lower your sodium intake. Tamari jōyu is made of soybeans, salt, and water. I recommend looking for organic, reduced sodium San-J brand tamari at your local health food store, major grocery store, or Japanese market. San-J tamari is made with all soybeans and no wheat for a richer flavor. Store, refrigerated, for up to one year.

Rice vinegar is a staple in Japanese households and it adds the perfect balance of flavors to each dish in this book. I'm a huge fan of kome su for its light and bright taste. Try it in your salad dressings, to finish off your marinades and sauces, or with a touch of citrus and soy sauce to make a homemade ponzu sauce. When purchasing, look for high-quality Japanese brands, like Marukan and Mitsukan (Mizkan).

sushi-su (sushi seasoning vinegar; 寿司酢, すしす): Sushi-su is simple rice seasoning made up of mostly rice vinegar, a touch of sugar, and a pinch of salt. This vinegar is used to season slightly cooled rice, to create a delicious sushi rice. You can find my recipe for sushi-su on page 167, or you can purchase it premade. Personally, I prefer the homemade version, and it's simple to whip up.

mirin (rice wine; 味醂, みりん): Mirin is Japanese rice wine used for cooking, which adds a delicious sweet flavor to many Japanese recipes. Look for brands that are made with quality ingredients (i.e., no high-fructose corn syrup) and are low in sugar. Mirin is delicious in sauces and dressings and can be used to deglaze your pans when cooking. You can also add it to your soups, or use it to finish or brighten a dish.

If you're looking to use a mirin that's not too sweet, I urge you to check out Hon Mirin (本みりん, ほんみりん), an authentic Japanese mirin made without any added sugar.

noodles

soba (蕎麦, そば): These Japanese-style buckwheat noodles, commonly used in Japanese broths, are served hot or cold. Soba noodles contain protein, fiber, and fewer calories than traditional pasta noodles made from refined wheat. I love cooking soba noodle soup, adding chilled soba to cold salads, and making *soba cha* (soba tea) with my Great-Auntie Takuko! You can find soba in most grocery stores.

udon (うどん): Commonly used in Japanese broth, udon are thick noodles made of only wheat flour, water, and salt. These thick and comforting noodles have an amazing, satisfying texture. Precooked (frozen or fresh) udon noodles cook up in no time and are simple to keep on hand in your freezer. The Japanese love their udon because they're considered an *oishii* (delicious!) comfort food for them. Check out page 113 for a yum udon recipe. You can find udon noodles at your local Japanese store. I recommend cooking with the precooked udon noodles found in the freezer or refrigerated sections versus dried udon.

fresh ramen noodles (ラーメン): Ramen are thin, commonly fried, wheat-based noodles; however, fresh varieties are available as well. Ramen is a serious Japanese comfort food, beloved by the whole country of Japan and all over the world. When purchasing dried ramen, ditch the salty, MSG-filled seasoning packet and instead cook the simple broth recipes in this book. I recommend buying quality fresh ramen, such as those from Sun Noodle brand, which you can find at your local Japanese store in the fridge or freezer section. See page 111 for my fave Spicy Miso-Tahini Ramen recipe!

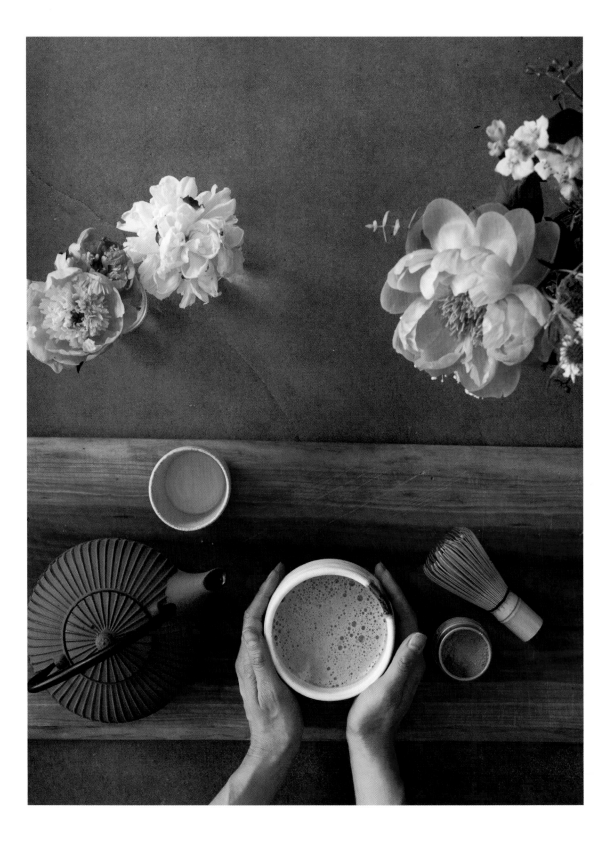

sōmen (素麺, そうめん): Sōmen are thin Japanese noodles, usually served cold and consumed in the hot summer months in Japan. Sōmen noodles are incredibly quick to cook—usually two to three minutes—and are a satisfying, delish complex carb. Look for these noodles at your local Japanese store.

green tea

matcha (green tea powder; 抹茶, まっちゃ): Originally enjoyed by Japanese monks and samurai, matcha is a finely milled green tea powder. Matcha is made of shade-grown, steamed tea leaves, which are ground into a top-quality green tea powder.

When you drink matcha, you are consuming the whole tea leaf. Thus, matcha is filled with more antioxidants, vitamin C, and L-theanine (which helps to promote relaxation and focus at the same time) than any other tea.

I make matcha with my *chasen* (bamboo whisk) and hot water (175° to 185°F) each morning, to stay focused on my work and slightly relaxed. Matcha should not be made with boiling water, but rather, water that has been boiled then slightly cooled. Matcha is additionally used in baking recipes and in some savory marinades and dressings. You'll find many here in this book. The Japanese love and prize traditional matcha tea ceremonies and their matcha tea cakes.

The quality of your matcha matters. Always look for the words *ceremonial grade* on the packaging, and opt for Japanese brands when purchasing. If the matcha powder is made in Japan, it will be ceremonial grade.

purchasing tea

When purchasing green tea, keep the following guidelines in mind:

- Buy and consume as needed—don't stockpile your teas.

- Look for green tea that is vibrant and bright in color, rather than brittle, dry, or dull in appearance.

- Be sure to store your green tea away from moisture, light, and heat. Store in an airtight container in a cool, dark, dry place.

- I've always believed that purchasing quality tea and foods is best. Purchase your tea from a reliable and reputable source with tea knowledge and quality control behind their product.

genmaicha (blend of rice and tea; 玄米茶, げんまいちゃ): This robust and umami-rich green tea is blended with roasted brown rice and is my favorite tea for steeping. Genmaicha is a special blend of two Japanese classics, roasted rice and sencha green tea. Most commonly it's a 50:50 blend, giving you that earthy, savory, roasted flavor. Genmaicha is perfect on a rainy day or just for a morning pick-me-up. Look for quality brands like Ito En or Yamamotoyama when purchasing.

sencha (green tea; 煎茶, せんちゃ): A must-have staple in Japanese households, sencha is a steamed Japanese green tea. It is the traditional classic green tea and, like all forms of green tea, contains high concentrations of EGCG (epigallocatechin gallate), a catechin that may help with optimal brain function and the prevention of cancer. Sencha tea leaves are steamed, dried, and rolled into a fine needlelike shape. Once infused in hot water, they can be steeped up to three times.

hōjicha (green tea; ほうじ茶): This roasted green tea is made from leaves that are darker in color from their roasting process. Hōjicha contains less caffeine than other varieties of green tea.

gyokuro (jade dew tea; 玉露, ぎょくろ): This is the queen of all green tea. It is shade-grown and beloved for its rich, sweet, umami flavor. Gyokuro also contains high levels of the amino acid L-theanine.

top-offs and flavor enhancers

goma (sesame seeds; 胡麻, ごま; and gomashio; ごま塩, ごましお): Goma refers to the whole sesame seed, and gomashio is a mixture of toasted and crushed sesame seeds flavored with sea salt, usually handmade in a Japanese *suribachi* (a Japanese-style mortar and pestle). You'll find that I sprinkle almost everything with goma or gomashio. Consider it my salt and pepper. I can't get enough of the earthy, nutty flavor and the extra boost of nutrients! Sesame seeds contain phytosterols, plant compounds that may help to reduce cholesterol. Gomashio is full of calcium, copper, phosphorus, zinc, and iron, minerals that all boost bone health.

katsuobushi (japanese dried bonito flakes; 鰹節, かつおぶし): Katsuobushi is dried, thinly shaved, sometimes fermented bonito flakes (from skipjack tuna or bonito). It is often used to make dashi (stock), to add bold umami flavor and seasoning to foods like gohan (hot cooked rice) and tofu, and to top off boiled spinach (*ohitashi*). Mom always told me the best onigiri (page 93) is made with soy sauce and katsuobushi placed into the middle! Katsuobushi is full of omega-3s, which help promote brain function. Store, tightly sealed in a resealable bag, in the fridge for up to one year.

furikake (ふりかけ): The best Japanese seasoning ever—I grew up putting this stuff on everything. Furikake is a Japanese mixed spice made up of toasted nori flakes, toasted sesame seeds, sometimes bonito flakes, dried fish, sometimes dried eggs, sugar, and salt. It comes in dozens of varieties and flavors, so be sure to check a few and find one you love. You can up the taste in just about anything with a touch of furikake.

karashi (japanese mustard; 辛子, からし): This hot Japanese mustard is my sister's favorite condiment. Japanese mustard has a spiciness much more potent than traditional American mustards, so a little goes a long way. Karashi comes in the form of paste or powder. This mustard is perfect when whipping up *nattō, oden,* and *shūmai.* Karashi is made of mustard seeds that contain phytonutrients that may help fight off cell mutation and tumors.

wasabi (わさび): Wasabi is one condiment you've definitely heard of, but it's not the kind you've been consuming at the sushi bar. True wasabi from Japan comes from the wasabi root, freshly grated and paired with sushi. Most "wasabi" consumed in the U.S. is horseradish with additives and color. True wasabi root is packed with vitamins and minerals, including magnesium, manganese, potassium, vitamin B_6, vitamin C, calcium, zinc, thiamine, phosphorus, copper, riboflavin, iron, folate, and niacin. You can find the real-deal wasabi at your local Japanese store. If you can't find fresh wasabi, opt for organic wasabi powder by Eden Foods. Store wasabi paste and powder in the fridge for up to one year (powder lasts for up to two years if refrigerated).

gari shōga (pickled ginger; がりしょうが) and shōga (ginger; 生姜 しょうが): The purest form of pickled ginger is its natural beige-ish color, not pink, so be selective when you purchase and opt for the natural stuff! Fresh ginger's antioxidants are a natural boost for your immune system. It is also an anti-inflammatory food that may alleviate pain and aid with digestion. In addition to eating it with sushi, I love finishing off my grain bowls with a few slices of pickled ginger.

shichimi tōgarashi (七味唐辛子, しちみとうがらし): This Japanese seven-spice mix is my favorite to add a little heat or a citrus boost to almost any dish. Tōgarashi is a popular Japanese spice blend made up of grated citrus peel, sanshō (Japanese pepper), dried chile, ginger, nori, black and white sesame seeds, and poppy seeds. The ingredients can vary. These anti-inflammatory ingredients contain capsaicin, which is known to strengthen your immune system and may clear congestion. Tōgarashi spice blend contains vitamins A, C, D, and E.

hoshi shiitake (dried shiitake mushrooms; 干し椎茸, ほししいたけ): A staple found in all Japanese households, dried shiitake mushrooms contain powerful, concentrated umami flavor. I love reconstituting them in water, using them in my soups and stir-fries, and saving the water they are soaked in to make delicious shiitake dashi. Shiitakes' B vitamins energize your body. They're also known for their beauty benefits, as shiitakes are high in selenium and zinc, which may help to clear your complexion. Sauté them with some toasted sesame oil, or add them to a soup, but don't overcook with moisture or they will become soggy! Purchase dried shiitakes at your local health food store or Japanese store and store tightly sealed in a cool, dark place for up to a year.

kiriboshi (dried daikon root; 切り干し大根, きりぼしだいこん): Daikon is a large white radish that is popular in Japan. *Daikon* means "big root" in Japanese, which is appropriate since daikon looks more like a root than a radish! Fresh daikon is often pickled but dried daikon is a kitchen staple in Japan that is often used in salads, soups, and stir-fries. It's a versatile ingredient that imparts earthiness and a slight sweetness to foods. Many Japanese home cooks use dried daikon year-round.

refrigerated basics

tofu (豆腐, とうふ): Tofu is a delicious, 100-percent vegan plant protein that my Japanese ancestors have been consuming for thousands of years. Made of soybean curds pressed into firm blocks, tofu is best purchased organic. It's also important to look for "non-GMO" labeling since so many of the soy crops are grown using GMO farming practices. Tofu is available in different varieties of firmness, including silken, medium, medium-firm, firm, extra-firm, baked, and savory.

Tofu is an inexpensive source of protein that is high in calcium, manganese, phosphorous, and selenium. It is additionally a great source of magnesium, copper, zinc, and energy-boosting vitamin B$_1$.

Top off your salads, stir-fries, and bowls with extra-firm tofu, or use silken tofu as a protein addition in any smoothie, dessert, or dressing.

miso paste (organic white, red, and *awase*; 味噌, みそ): Miso is a delicious umami paste made from fermented soybeans, *kōji* (*Aspergillus oryzae*), water, and salt. Miso paste comes in three basic varieties: white (*shiro*); red (*aka*); and *awase*, a mix of white and red. Purchase and cook with miso to your taste preference. The darker the miso, the more intense the flavor. Think of miso like craft beer—the lighter the color, the milder the taste. The darker the color the deeper the flavor. Texturally, miso paste can either be smooth or slightly chunky.

Next to soy sauce, miso is, in my opinion, is the most versatile ingredient in Japanese cuisine. I use it daily to make soups, marinades, dressings, dips, reductions, and glazes. Miso is typically cooked in savory Japanese dishes, but can be used in some sweet treats. You can also add a touch of miso to your avocados (as a snack), pasta, mac 'n' cheese, soba noodles, or grain bowls. I've gotten so many of my girlfriends hooked on miso, they now take photos and send me their most amazing creations. Miso love! Because miso is fermented, it offers probiotic benefits, which may help to boost immunity and brain health as well as digestive health. Miso is also full of B vitamins, vitamin K, protein, fiber, antioxidants, copper, zinc, and omega-3 fats.

Other grains like barley (*mugi miso*) and rice (*kome miso*) are sometimes fermented to make miso in Japan. In the U.S. I've seen everything from quinoa to pumpkin used to make small-batch miso.

The process of fermenting miso can take up to one year, sometimes longer, sometimes shorter. When purchasing, opt for organic and non-GMO varieties.

saikyō miso (西京みそ, さいきょうみそ): A sweet miso paste originally made in Kyoto, saikyō miso is from a combination of fermented rice and soybeans, with a higher ratio of rice to soybeans. This variety of miso is often used in soups, glazes, and marinades for lighter fare such as veggies and fish dishes.

umeboshi (pickled plums; 梅干, うめぼし): Umeboshi, also known as *ume*, is a small, sour, and salty Japanese plum, similar to a tiny apricot. These tart, delicious pickled plums contain iron, calcium, and phosphorus, and are high in pectin, which may aid in digestion.

The Japanese use natural red/purple shiso (perilla) leaves for the natural pale red coloring of umeboshi. In fact, a traditional Japanese bentō rice box can be topped off with one single umeboshi plum in the middle, making it a symbolic Japanese flag! Umeboshi plums can be found in the refrigerated aisle of your Japanese market. Look for natural varieties that don't contain dyes.

adzuki (adzuki beans; 小豆, あずき): These small, powerful red beans are packed with antioxidants, protein, iron, zinc, magnesium, potassium, and, of course, fiber. Adzuki beans, also known as *aduki* beans, may

Okinawa, Japan: The varieties of tofu and miso are endless.

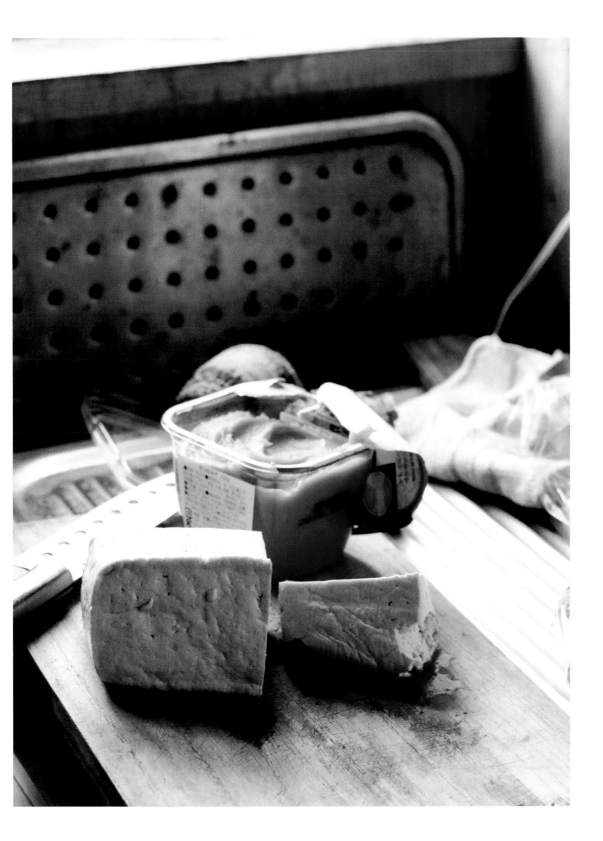

fermented foods every day, the Japanese way

Here's a simple philosophy to follow: Eat something fermented every day. After studying in Japan the past few years, I noticed my skin improved, my nails became stronger, my hair grew faster, and my digestion was much more regular. I believe that these changes were due in part to the large amount of fermented foods I ate each day.

Fermented foods contain bacteria that help to promote gut health, and your gut health is linked to everything from your immunity to your mood (some research even suggests it can help protect against depression). When you give the healthy bacteria in your gut a little probiotic boost, they can help the body digest and absorb the essential vitamins and nutrients you need for optimal health.

My favorite fermented foods include miso paste, reduced-sodium soy sauce and tamari, umeboshi plums, kombucha tea, nattō, tempeh (fermented soybeans, similar to tofu), tsukemono (Japanese pickles), and rice vinegar. If you aren't able to eat fermented foods daily, I recommend taking a vegan probiotic supplement to get a similar benefit.

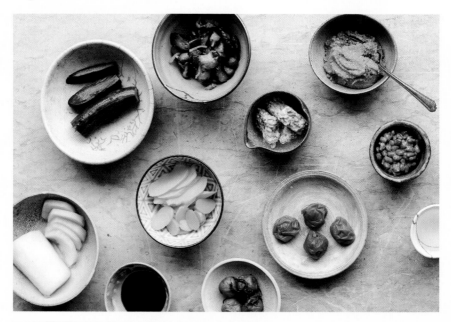

help with heart health and maintaining a healthy weight. The Japanese consume adzuki beans both savory and sweet, hot and cold. They are used in the popular macrobiotic eating style and are considered to be a prized superfood. My favorite ways to enjoy adzuki beans? Sweet adzuki mochi, dango with adzuki, and adzuki over shaved ice. Savory wise, I love adzuki beans in my bowls, *sekihan*, and macrobiotic salads. You can purchase adzuki beans canned (drain and rinse well) or dried (soak and simmer in water, drain). Once you've opened the can or rehydrated the dried beans, store them tightly sealed in the fridge for up to one week.

fresh produce

ginger (shōga; 生姜, しょうが): Potent, and full of anti-inflammatory compounds, this rhizome from the ginger plant is commonly found in Japanese cuisine and is usually grated, ground, or finely sliced and added to marinades, stir-fries, dressings, and sauces.

turmeric (ukon; ウコン): Magical turmeric, also a rhizome, has a pungent taste and a bright yellow color. Turmeric has been used in Okinawan households for centuries (Okinawans love their fermented turmeric tea!) and it's speculated that this practice has contributed to the legendary Okinawan longevity. Turmeric has many anti-inflammatory properties and has been shown to help prevent cancer, fight arthritis pain, and support cognitive health.

Turmeric is typically used in Japanese curry dishes (Japanese curry is slightly different from the Indian and Thai curries you may be accustomed to, as it's not made with coconut milk). Lucky for you, I've added turmeric to several recipes in this book, including a Turmeric-Kale Fried Rice (page 132) I think you will love.

shiitake mushroom (shiitake; 椎茸, しいたけ): Commonly used in Japanese cuisine, fresh and dried shiitake mushrooms are a staple in Japanese households. These beauties are some of the most overlooked of all superfoods, and I encourage each of you to start cooking with shiitakes! You'll find fresh shiitake mushrooms throughout this book. You can always cook with shiitake mushrooms in place of any meat. Look for firm, fresh, bounce-back-to-the-touch mushrooms, and store them in your refrigerator. When fresh isn't an option, dried shiitakes work as well (see page 55).

daikon (large japanese radish; 大根, だいこん): Daikon can be eaten ground, pickled, shaved, boiled, or roasted in soups, stir-fries, and salads. Daikon is packed with fiber, potassium, and vitamin C and is very low in calories. A total superfood, daikon is also known to be a natural diuretic. Look for these gorgeous, large radishes at your local market. Make sure the flesh is white, with no bruising (a touch of green is okay), and ones with green leaves attached are even better (you can cook the leaves too!). Store in the refrigerator for up to a week.

kabocha squash (南瓜, かぼちゃ): Quite possibly one of my favorite foods, kabocha squash, when cooked, is buttery, nutty, and sweet. Most Japanese consume kabocha with its simple-to-eat green skin left on. I love kabocha cooked up in soup, roasted and tossed into my salads, and the traditional Japanese way, in *Kabocha no Nitsuke Shōyu Aji* (page 163), a recipe my mom showed me how to make in Kyūshū. Kabocha is packed with beta-carotene, iron, potassium, fiber, vitamin C, and even protein. Make sure to look for a firm and gorgeous kabocha squash (it looks like a flat, round, green pumpkin), usually available in the fall and winter months.

green onions/scallions (negi; ねぎ): The Japanese love their green onions, which are used to top off a variety of dishes like miso soup, stir-fries, soba, udon, ramen, and *gyōza*. You'll find them all over this book, so do keep in mind their magical benefits. Green onions are packed with immunity-boosting benefits and vitamins C and K.

napa cabbage (hakusai; 白菜, はくさい): I use this delicious, crisp cabbage in many of my recipes, such as *donabe*, *sukiyaki*, salads, and soups, and it is often made into delicious kimchi. Napa cabbage has a distinct white rib and a beautiful light green leaf on top. It is rich in folic acid and vitamins K and C. It's also a natural diuretic and an immunity booster, making it a great choice to consume in the colder months.

bunashimeji (shimeji mushrooms; ぶなしめじ, しめじ): These mushrooms, which come in a cute tiny little bunch, are also known as beech mushrooms. They are in season year-round and may only be found at Japanese supermarkets. Bunashimeji mushrooms contain B and D vitamins and are a seriously delish way to get more zinc and copper. I personally love cooking these juicy, flavorful mushrooms in my soups, with soba noodles, and in sautés for an extra hit of umami. When purchasing mushrooms, look for firm and fresh mushrooms by pressing lightly on them. Hokto is a reputable and reliable brand for mushrooms in the U.S.

spinach (hōrensō; ほうれん草,ほうれんそう): The Japanese love their spinach, and adding a handful of fresh spinach to soups and other hot dishes is one of the quickest and easiest ways to add more nutrients to your bowl! Spinach is a major source of magnesium, potassium, folate, iron, calcium, and vitamins A, C, and K. I add spinach to all my smoothies for a daily hit of green nutrients. Look for fresh, perky, unwilted green leaves. You can save some cash by purchasing whole-leaf spinach in a bunch, versus baby spinach—just be sure to wash it thoroughly before using! Unwashed, it will keep in the fridge for about a week.

burdock root (gobō; 牛蒡, ごぼう): Burdock root, also known as gobō root, may help to reduce the risk of heart disease and aids in maintaining healthy blood pressure. Gobō is high in potassium and can help to keep your skin hydrated and glowing. It's high in fiber and inulin, which keep your tummy happy. Gobō root may help the body to flush toxins. And gobō, high in vitamins C and E, can boost your immunity.

The Japanese love eating gobō stir-fried and pickled, and I use it in my *kakiage* (mixed tempura). I grew up eating delicious gobō root and will never forget my mom making her delicious *kinpira gobō* (page 91). You can find the long, thin, dark-colored burdock root at health food stores or Japanese food stores.

be open to new, nourishing inspiration

shōjin ryōri
精進料理, しょうじんりょうり,
food of the monks, devotional cuisine

Shōjin ryōri is the devotional cuisine of monks in Japan. The purpose of shōjin ryōri is to celebrate seasonal vegetables, to nourish, to utilize all the parts of the plants, to energize and enlighten, and to cook and eat with harmony and peace. No potent flavors, such as onions or garlic, are included in these meals, and no animal products are used.

These days it's easy to forget that veganism and vegetarianism aren't food trends that started in the '60s—they have been a philosophy and way of life for many people in many cultures since the thirteenth century.

While staying at a local temple with monks in the mountains in Kōyasan, my sister and I ate and studied shōjin ryōri, which completely changed the way I cook and eat today. I learned to use more plant-based foods, to work with veggies, fruits, whole grains, fermented foods, and plant-based proteins. These are the kinds of foods that, I've come to learn, work in harmony with my body and mind and that make me feel good.

The recipes in this book are mostly seasonal and plant-based, designed to make you feel lighter, more vibrant, happier, and healthier. I'm so excited to share shōjin ryōri with you. It is not a diet—it is heritage, culture, tradition (mixed with some modernization), and a way of life.

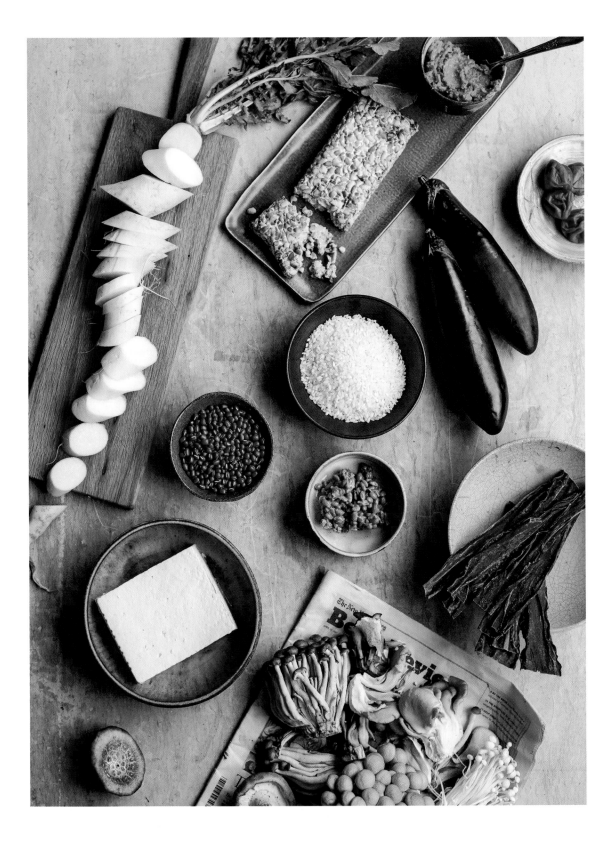

basics used in shōjin ryōri

The basis for shōjin ryōri meals is gohan (rice; ご飯, ごはん).

The Japanese enjoy a small amount of rice with just about every meal. We usually cook short-grain white rice, as rice helps to satiate your appetite and balance your meals. White rice is a good source of iron, protein, and vitamin B_1. There is much history found in these polished grains. Long ago, making white rice took excess time and labor (not as simple as we have it now!).

In the old days, white rice was consumed only by those who were wealthy and of high class. My mom explained to me, "We offer white rice to gods and Buddha, but now the present-day economy is so much better and technology is so advanced that everybody can enjoy white rice." White rice reminds us all that there is history in each of the foods we eat—and that it is important to have gratitude for what we have.

Additional components of these traditional meals include:

Tofu

Seasonal and local vegetables

Dried vegetables

Miso

Seaweed

Mushrooms

Beans

Tea

Umeboshi plums

As I became more and more interested in cooking *washoku*, the traditional meals of Japan, I knew it was time to educate myself on the traditions of my heritage. My best teachers were my Okaasan (mom), Baachan grandma), my Great-Auntie Takuko, my friends Yukari Sakamoto and Rona Tison, and my sensei Elizabeth Andoh. I've learned so much from them that I want to share with you. Here is a brief overview of some of the key concepts of traditional Japanese cuisine.

washoku; 和食

The term *washoku* refers to the deep-rooted traditional and regional cuisine of Japan. *Wa* 和 translates to "Japan/harmony/peace" and *shoku* 食 translates to "eat" or "food." Instead of just practicing a plant-based diet, my goal for you is to feel more connected to and in harmony with your nutrition. You will experience the subtle and simple flavors the Japanese use in their traditional recipes. You'll learn the artful balance of sweet, savory, sour, small amounts of fat, and deep umami flavor. We will also be cooking with plenty of fresh produce, just as Mom taught me back in California. Nourish your beautiful mind and spirit with the harmonious art of washoku! (Note that while some of these recipes are traditional, many are also adapted to an American-style palate or what is accessible to us in the States.)

hara hachi bu; 腹八分, はらはちぶ

The Japanese idea of *hara hachi bu* means to eat only until you are 80 percent full. It's not about deprivation, but rather satisfaction and moderation. Never eating until you feel "full" means you'll never feel uncomfortably *too* full. Try it by practicing eating just until you feel satiated. You'll feel lighter, you'll have more energy, and your digestion will improve!

umami; 味 旨味 うまみ

Umami is the "fifth taste" (after sweet, salty, acidic, and bitter), a savory flavor which can best be described as earthy. The Japanese incorporate an umami element into every dish. Some Japanese chefs believe that umami is so powerful, it is the "healthy" foundation of Japanese cuisine. Common sources of umami include mushrooms, soy sauce, and miso.

itadakimasu! いただきます!

The term *Itadakimasu* means "I am receiving this meal, thank you." It is said prior to eating each meal in Japan. This ritual is meant to pay respect and offer appreciation for the food you are going to eat—you are thanking everyone who partook in creating the meal, and honoring your own ability to receive that meal. Before each meal, practice saying enthusiastically to yourself and others you are dining with "Itadakimasu!"

kaiseki-ryōri; 会席料理 / 懐石料理 かいせきりょうり

Two Chinese characters are used for kaiseki-ryōri.

1. 会席 is used for first-class cuisine/traditional Japanese banquets.
2. 懐石 is used for a simple meal served before a tea ceremony; it can also mean a first-class refined cuisine served before a tea ceremony.

Traditionally, kaiseki-ryōri was a simple meal served before a tea ceremony. Hundreds of years later, it has evolved into a formal, beautifully plated meal, eaten with others and adjusted to your liking. You may see the term *kaiseki-ryōri* on a menu at a Japanese restaurant. It refers to a meal of the chef's choice of seasonal, small plates. It's easy to make your own kaiseki- or bentō-style meals at home—just choose two to five recipes, use your best plates, and enjoy with good friends.

moritsuke; 盛り付け, もりつけ

The Japanese love to eat with their eyes! Traditionally, the Japanese prefer beautiful, detailed, small plates to share a wide variety of colorful and nutritious eats with the family. The term *moritsuke* refers to Japanese beauty plating. The Japanese also love their small plates to keep a variety of food separate. It's a super-Westernized custom to serve all the components of one meal on a large plate. The Japanese believe that if you make food look enticing, beautiful, and delicious, you and your family will be more inclined to eat healthy, fresh, and nutritious foods.

We like to make bentō boxes *fun* and creative, especially for kids, so they can explore and try new foods and enjoy mealtimes. You'll often see rice molded into animals or faces, little pickles, and fruit cut into playful shapes. You'll see my favorites in my kawaii bentō box on page 141.

gochisōsama deshita; ご馳走様でした, ごちそうさまでした

The Japanese term *gochisōsama deshita* refers to the ritual of closing and expressing gratitude for a delicious meal. Generally speaking, the term is directed toward the person/people who cooked and made the meal. The term also pays tribute and respect to the farmers, the grocers, and the laborers who all took part in helping to get the meal to the table. It is a beautiful and honorable way to tell everyone, "Thank you for this meal, I am grateful for all, I am satisfied and finished, it was delicious!" It is one of my all-time favorite Japanese rituals.

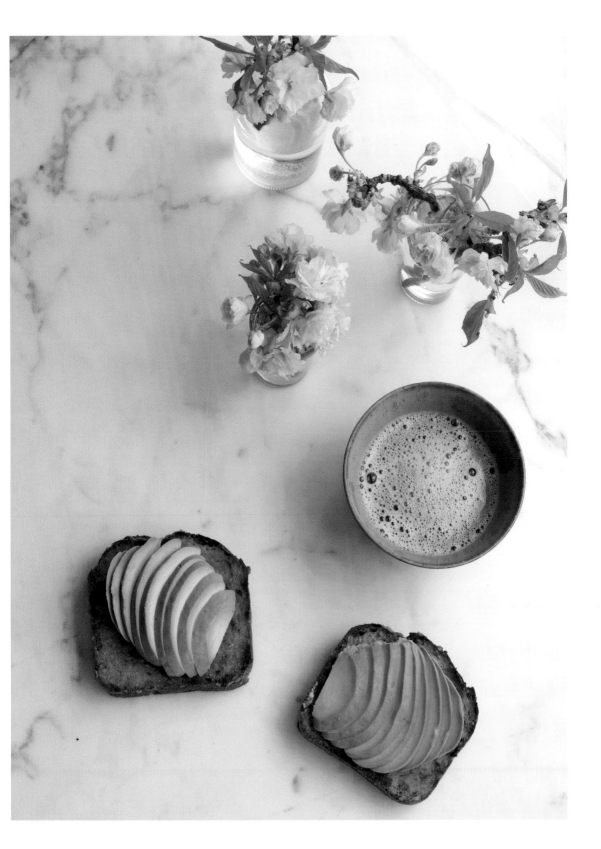

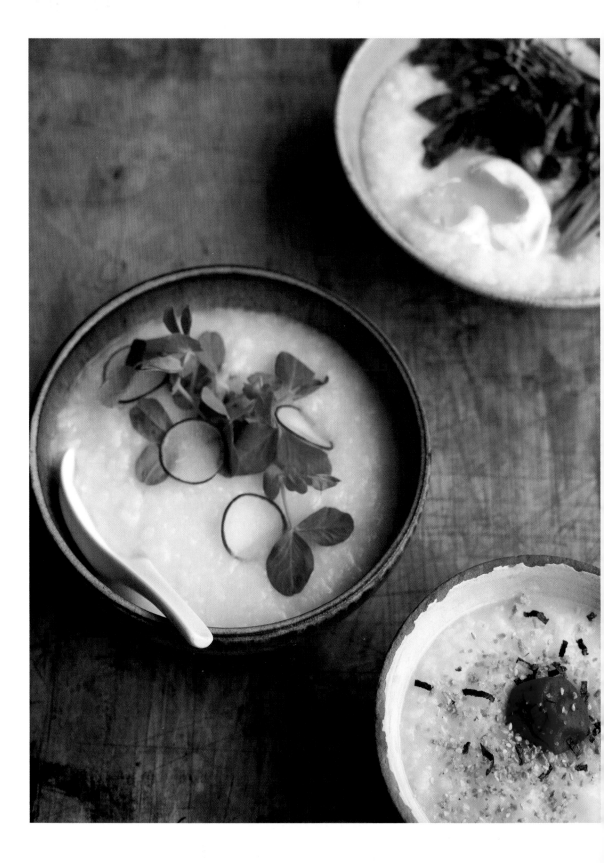

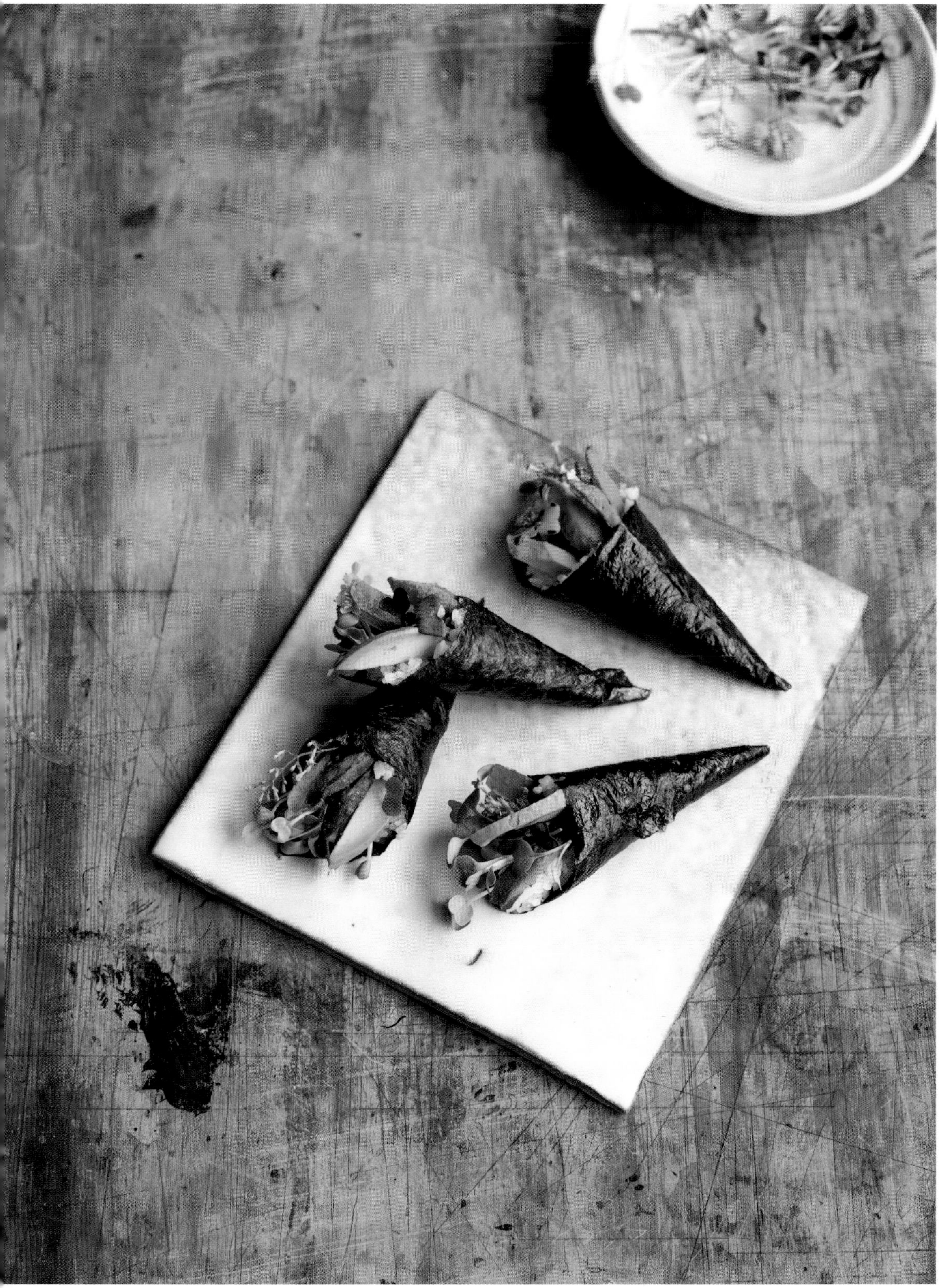

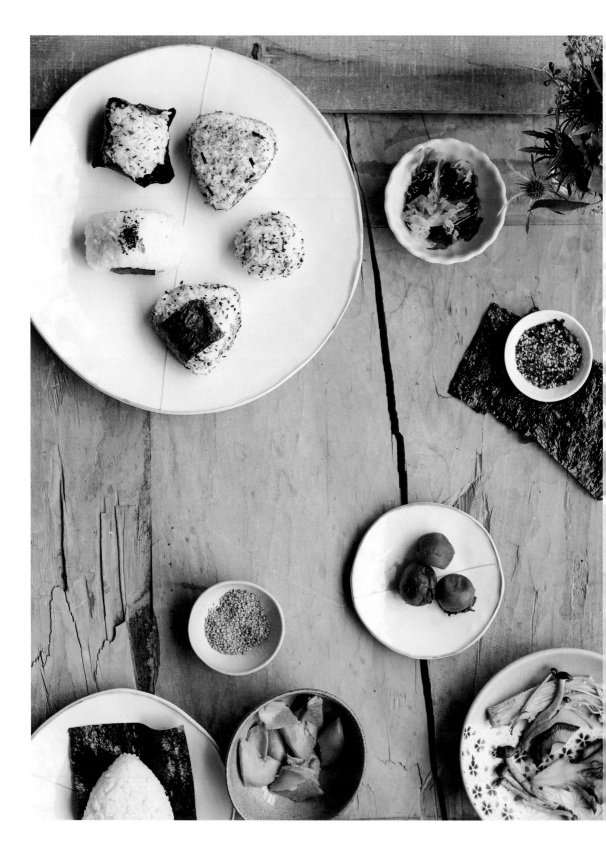

breakfast & starters

朝ご飯，あさごはん

asa gohan

matcha-coconut love smoothie

Serves 2

This matcha-coconut pick-me-up is the perfect morning meal! With a boost of spinach plus matcha, you'll feel nourished from the day's start. For extra energy add a scoop of your favorite plant-based protein powder.

1 cup unsweetened coconut water or almond milk

2 cups organic baby spinach

½ frozen banana

2 teaspoons high-quality matcha green tea powder

1 tablespoon unsweetened dried coconut flakes, or ½ cup fresh coconut pieces

½ cup ice, if desired

Put all the ingredients into a high-powered blender and blend until smooth. Serve immediately.

sweet potato–cinnamon smoothie

Serves 3 or 4

This simple and nutritious sweet potato smoothie reminds me of my friends in Okinawa! Use leftover baked or roasted sweet potatoes to create this delicious and creamy smoothie that's brimming with beauty-savvy nutrients vitamin A and beta-carotene, plus a boost of fiber to fill you up.

2 cups leftover mashed or roasted sweet potatoes (see Note)

½ teaspoon ground cinnamon

1½ cups unsweetened almond milk

1 cup light coconut milk

1 cup ice

Put all the ingredients into a high-powered blender and blend until smooth. Serve immediately.

NOTE

To make roasted sweet potatoes, peel two sweet potatoes and cut them into 1-inch cubes. Toss with coconut oil and roast at 350°F for 38 to 40 minutes. Cool before blending.

japanese rice porridge

okayu お粥, おかゆ

Serves 6

Okayu is a Japanese rice porridge that is a simple and inexpensive way to fill your tummy. A comforting dish for the Japanese, it's often made with chicken stock to help someone heal from a cold. Okayu can also be made with the leftover soup from a nabe pot or miso. This filling and delicious porridge keeps well in the fridge for days.

2 cups uncooked medium-grain white rice, rinsed and drained

7 to 8 cups purified water, dashi (see page 117), or stock/broth

Two 5-inch pieces kombu or wakame

Avocado slices, katsuobushi, shōyu (soy sauce), miso, arugula, and/or tōgarashi, for topping (optional)

Put the rinsed rice into a large stockpot. Add the water or stock (for a thick porridge, add 7 cups of the water; for a thinner porridge, add all 8 cups water) add your kombu pieces and cook the rice over medium heat for about 15 minutes.

Reduce the heat to medium-low and cook for 15 minutes more, stirring occasionally. Continue to cook, stirring, until the rice has absorbed all the water and is cooked through.

Ladle the porridge into six individual serving bowls. Garnish and enjoy!

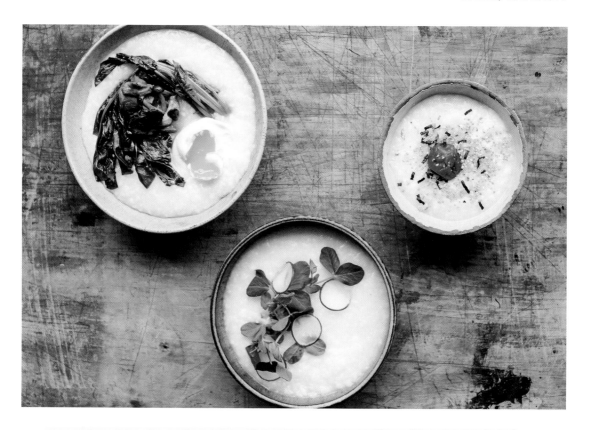

japanese mom knows best
different ways to enjoy okayu!

Okayu has a similar reputation to chicken soup in the United States; it's the go-to dish to serve and eat when you're feeling under the weather. Here my mom shares two alternative and creative ways to enjoy okayu as a healing and comfort food. Don't wait for the sniffles to try them!

zōsui; 雑炊 ぞうすい: Okayu + vegetables: Cook in a nabe (short for "donabe") pot; add salt to simply season!

chagayu; 茶粥 ちゃがゆ: Chagayu is gohan cooked with tea instead of water. In this version, you boil the rice in roasted green tea, for a true, light, umami finish. As Mom says, "So yum!"

traditional japanese breakfast

miso + gohan + tsukemono みそ＋ごはん＋つけもの

Serves 4 for breakfast (but can be customized; see below)

A traditional Japanese breakfast is made up of hot gohan (rice), tsukemono (Japanese pickles), miso shiru (miso soup), and the occasional tamago kake gohan (hot steamy rice with an egg cracked on top) or tamagoyaki (Japanese omelet).

Here's everything you'll need for a satisfying Japanese breakfast for four. Adjust the quantities according to party size (see photo for reference).

4 cups cooked gohan (white rice), still hot

4 cups miso soup (easy miso soup with root veggies, see page 102)

Tsukemono (Japanese pickles)

1 tamagoyaki (Japanese omelet, see page 152) or other protein (optional)

Serve up four bowls of hot steamy white rice.

Serve up four bowls of hot miso soup.

Serve pickles in small plates.

Plate up your favorite proteins, as you'd like: tamagoyaki, salmon, tofu.

Add your favorite Japanese condiments at the table: furikake, karashi, shōyu, etc.

Itadakimasu!

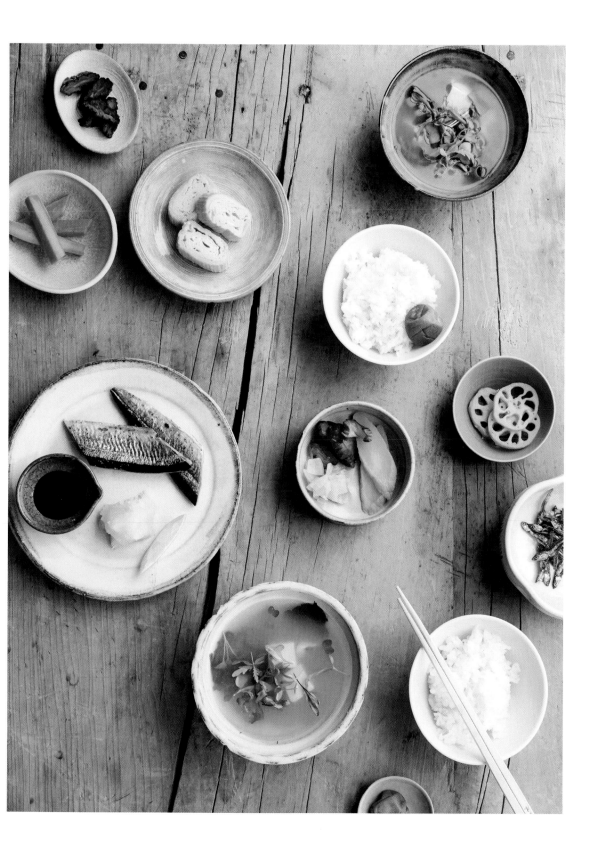

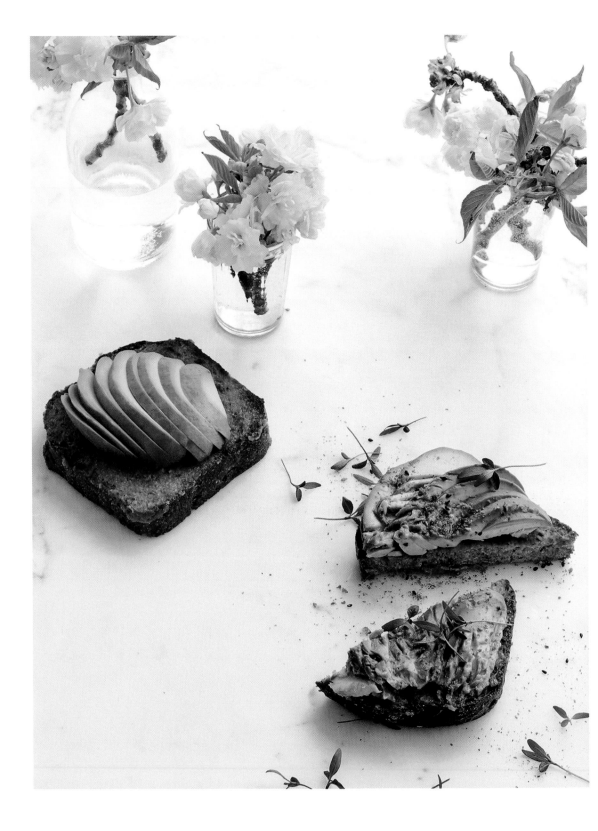

miso avocado toast

Serves 2

The first time I tested this recipe, I ate it three times in one day, for each meal of the day. That should tell you something about how delicious this umami-rich version of avocado toast is! The combo of miso and avocado seems obvious to me now; I can't believe I'd never tried it before. This dish comes together in minutes and will seriously up your avo-toast game.

Coconut oil or olive oil cooking spray, for the skillet

2 slices of your favorite bread

4 teaspoons organic red or white miso paste

1 ripe avocado, pitted, peeled, and thinly sliced

Pinch of tōgarashi

Pinch of gomashio

Toast the bread: Coat a medium skillet with cooking spray and place over medium heat. Add the bread slices to the skillet and toast on both sides, 1 to 2 minutes per side.

Slather a small amount of miso paste on one side of each slice of bread. Lightly spray the pan with extra cooking spray to prevent sticking. Return the toast to the pan, miso-side down, for just a minute or two, until lightly golden.

Remove the toast from the skillet and transfer to a clean work surface, miso-side up. Top with avocado slices and mash with a fork, if desired.

Sprinkle with tōgarashi and/or gomashio, and serve immediately.

furikake popcorn

Serves 4 to 6 as a snack or appetizer

This simple snack is perfect as an appetizer before a Japanese-style dinner party, or just for a relaxing movie night in.

¾ cup organic popcorn kernels (purchase in the bulk section)

1 to 2 tablespoons coconut oil, melted, or extra-virgin olive oil

4 to 5 tablespoons furikake

¼ teaspoon sea salt

Organic coconut oil or olive oil spray (if you'd like more coated popcorn)

Place the organic popcorn kernels into a medium brown bag. Fold the top down to close. Pop in the microwave for about 2 minutes on a normal setting, or until you begin to hear only a few kernels popping with 3 seconds between each pop, toward the end. Be sure to monitor popping to avoid burning.

Carefully remove the bag from the microwave and add the melted coconut oil or olive oil, furikake, and sea salt. Shake well to combine. If you need more coating for the furikake, spray lightly with organic coconut or olive oil spray and gently toss in the bag again.

tempura,
天麩羅 天ぷら, てんぷら

Making tempura at home is a lot easier than you think! You'll need a large deep pan, some frying oil, and the perfect combination of flour, water, and egg.

A sprinkle of Maldon or another coarse sea salt at the end to finish will make all the difference! Serve with a side of homemade tempura dipping sauce (page 89).

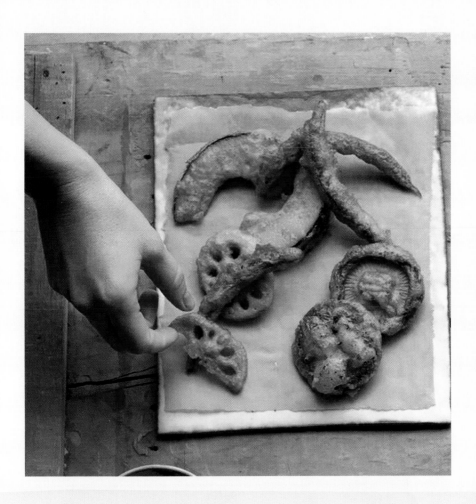

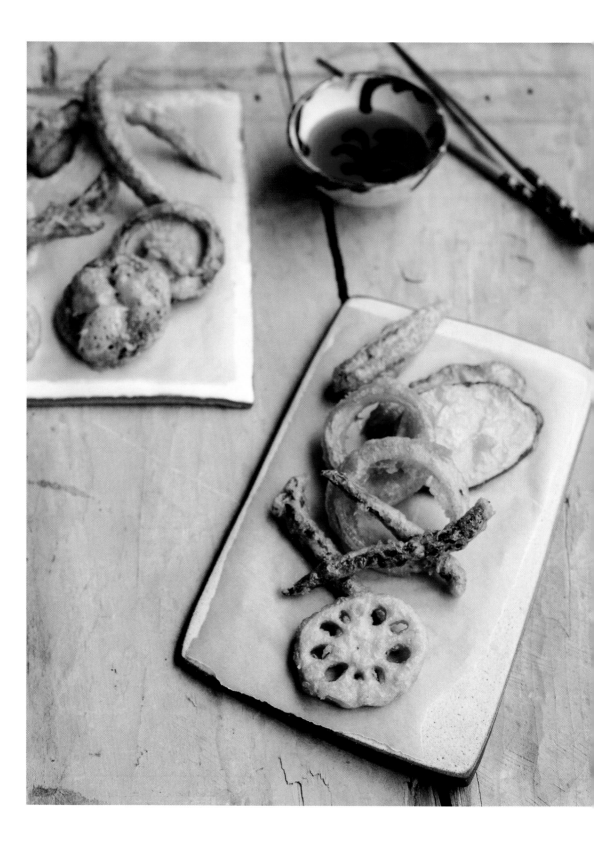

veggie tempura
野菜の天ぷら、やさい の てんぷら

Serves 4 to 6 as an appetizer

Fresh veggies, battered and deep-fried into crisp tempura and dipped in tempura sauce is everything in Japan. It's always okay to find balance in your lifestyle. I've learned from the Japanese that as long as you are active and living a healthy lifestyle, you can always indulge. Try this recipe out as a weekend treat and share with your friends!

TEMPURA

4 cups rice bran oil (kome abura); (see sidebar)

1 cup cake flour

1 large egg

1¼ cups ice-cold water or seltzer water

1 teaspoon baking soda

1 teaspoon cornstarch

Maldon or other sea salt, for finishing

VEGGIES

(Approximately 10 cups of your choice of veggies)

Sweet potatoes, skin-on, thinly sliced into disks

Kabocha squash, unpeeled, thinly sliced into half-moons

Green beans, trimmed

Shiitake mushrooms, whole, stems removed

Onions, sliced into rings

Large carrots, peeled, sliced

Burdock root, shaved, peeled, thinly sliced on the bias

Lotus root, sliced

Okra, top trimmed, sliced

2 tablespoons cake flour, for lightly tossing the veggies in before deep frying

You can find rice bran oil, or *kome abura* (米油 こめゆ, こめあぶら), also known as *kome yu*, at your local Japanese grocery store. You can also substitute vegetable oil for deep-frying, if necessary.

Line a large baking sheet with paper towels.

In a large bowl, combine the veggies of your choice and toss lightly with 2 tablespoons of the cake flour.

In a large pot, carefully heat the oil over medium-high heat.

In a separate medium bowl, add remaining tempura ingredients together and whisk until combined to make batter. Grab a small handful of the flour-coated veggies and carefully dredge them in the tempura batter, lightly coating them. Carefully lower the batter-coated veggies into the hot oil and fry.

When the veggies are golden brown and float to the top, use a slotted spoon, spider, or chopsticks to carefully transfer them to the prepared baking sheet to drain excess oil. Serve up with tempura sauce (see page 89), or spicy mayo. See page 90 for a picture of kakiage.

tempura reheating and storage

Tempura is best served when fresh and hot. Always use a paper towel to drain any excess oil. If you have leftover tempura, store it in a paper towel–lined, airtight container in the fridge for up to a week. To reheat, bring the tempura to room temperature. Place the tempura into a hot pan and reheat on both sides until slightly warmed through. Or you can preheat the oven to 375°F and reheat your room-temperature tempura on a baking sheet just until warmed through, 5 to 6 minutes.

kakiage かき揚げ, かきあげ

Serves 4 as an appetizer

This super-crisp and thinly sliced tempura treat is a Japanese household favorite when you've got leftover veggies to use up! My Japanese friends love kakiage (crisp tempura-battered and fried veggie cakes) as a once-in-a-while treat. This recipe is best paired with my fave umami-style tempura sauce, or a spicy vegan sriracha mayo for dipping! YUM!

VEGGIES (Can be any leftovers you have, too!)

2 medium carrots or sweet potatoes, julienned (or you can mix it up!)

2 cups shiitake mushrooms (stems removed), sliced, or try breaking up enoki or maitake mushrooms

1 yellow onion, thinly sliced

1 medium burdock root, thinly shaved

¼ kabocha squash, unpeeled, thinly sliced into strips

2 tablespoons cake flour, for dusting the veggies

TEMPURA

4 cups rice bran oil (kome abura) for deep frying

1 large egg

1¼ cups ice cold water

1 teaspoon aluminum-free baking soda

1 cup cake flour

High-quality sea salt, such as Maldon, for finishing

TEMPURA DIPPING SAUCE
(Cook all together over a medium-low heat, for about 10 minutes.)

¼ cup mirin

1 cup dashi (page 117)

2 tablespoons reduced-sodium, organic tamari soy sauce

Prepare a paper towel–lined sheet tray, set asisde.

In a large bowl, combine all the thinly sliced veggies and toss lightly with the 2 tablespoons cake flour; do not overmix.

In a large pot, over medium-high heat, carefully heat the oil until hot.

In a separate bowl, whisk remaining tempura ingredients together, well.

With one clean hand, scoop $1/3$ cup of the thinly sliced veggie mix, and lightly coat the shaved veggies in the batter (hold the veggies together as firmly as possible).

Carefully place each $1/3$ cup of the battered veggies into the hot oil to fry into a small kakiage cake. When golden brown and floating to the top, remove and place on a paper towel–lined sheet tray to remove any excess oil.

Continue until all batter is gone and pair with the dipping sauce to serve!

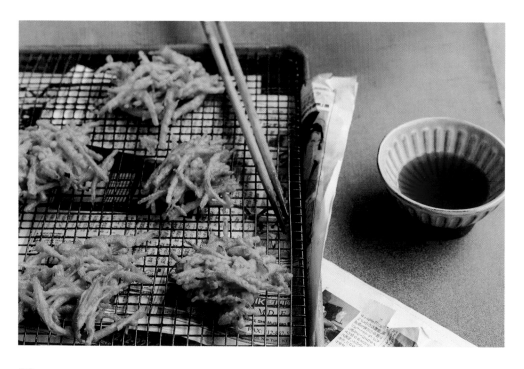

stir-fried burdock root kinpira gobō,
金平牛蒡 きんぴらごぼう

Serves as a side or as an entrée with rice

Burdock root is a fiber-loaded veggie with a firm and chewy texture. To me, it tastes a bit like an earthier version of a sunchoke mixed with sweet carrots. Be sure to serve this recipe with gohan (hot steamy rice), as kinpira gobō is salty!

1 medium carrot

1 medium burdock root (gobō)

1 tablespoon extra-virgin olive oil

2 teaspoons organic sugar (Mom's tip: you can also use mirin!)

2½ tablespoons reduced-sodium tamari soy sauce

1 tablespoon toasted sesame oil

1 tablespoon toasted sesame seeds

Cut the carrot into thin 2-inch-long julienne strips.

Wash and scrub (don't peel) the burdock root. Shave the burdock: Score/shave from the thicker end of the root to the thinner end, using a knife or a veggie peeler. Once peeled, slice the burdock into thin 2-inch-long julienne strips as you did the carrot.

In a medium sauté pan, warm the olive oil over medium-high heat. Add the carrot and burdock to the pan, lower the heat to medium, and stir-fry until fragrant, about 10 minutes.

Add the sugar and stir-fry for about 2 minutes more, until the sugar melts. Add the soy sauce and keep stirring until the liquid has evaporated, 1 to 2 minutes. Add the sesame oil and sesame seeds and stir to coat the veggies. Turn off the heat and enjoy immediately over a bowl of rice or as a side dish.

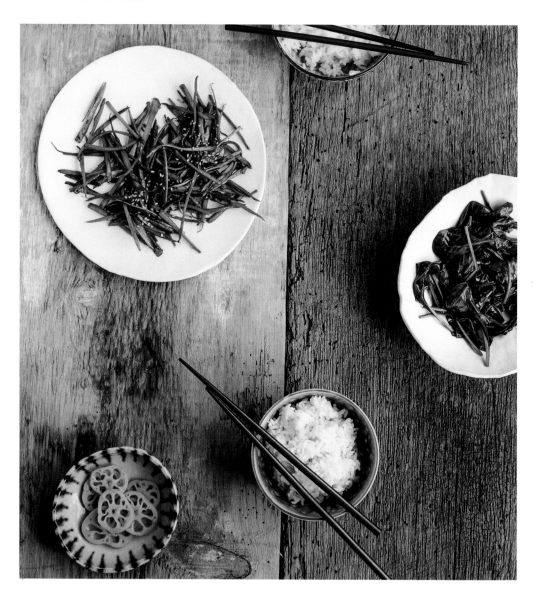

onigiri おにぎり

Serves 6 to 8

This recipe is nostalgia and childhood memories, all wrapped up in nori. My mother was always the most beautiful to me when she was cooking. She was quiet and focused, and she was living in the moment. Onigiri is a childhood treat that I took with me everywhere. My Japanese friends and family love taking them to the park for a lunch or snack on the go. Onigiri is about customizing your meal or snack. You can keep it vegan with umeboshi, takuan (pickles), avocado, sweet potato, and mushrooms, or you can add a protein like salmon. You make them however you want! Below are a few of my favorite suggestions.

3 U.S. cups cooked and slightly cooled rice (1½ cups uncooked rice, washed) (see sidebar, page 000)

⅓ cup lukewarm water

Salt

2 or 3 sheets nori, folded and torn into squares. Fold in half, then fold again into quarters, to make 10 to 12 squares. Press creases firmly and tear nori sheets along lines.

Toasted gomashio or furikake, for coating (optional)

TRADITIONAL JAPANESE FILLINGS
Umeboshi plums or umeboshi paste

Tsukemono (Japanese pickles)

Katsuobushi (Japanese dried bonito flakes)

Salted salmon (cooked salmon with a touch of salt and pepper, Mom's recipe!)

Shiitake mushrooms, cooked with sesame seeds, mirin and soy sauce

NONTRADITIONAL FILLINGS
Avocado mixed with mayo and sriracha

Roasted sweet potato pieces, tossed in miso, and sriracha

OISHII CREATIVE FILLINGS
Sautéed sliced mushrooms with avocado

Avocado cubes with a touch of soy sauce and roasted carrots

In a rice cooker, or a large pot, cook the rice to perfection. Remove from the heat and set aside to cool. If using a rice cooker: use $1^1/_2$ cups uncooked (rinsed) rice and 3 cups water and cook until hot and steamy.

Pour the lukewarm water into a small bowl and add a pinch of salt. Wet your hands with the water, so the rice won't stick.

Place ¼ cup/scoop of the slightly cooled rice on one hand, flatten it, and place your choice of fillings (umeboshi, avocado, tsukemono, cooked mushrooms, etc.) in the middle of the rice. Cover it with another ¼ cup/ scoop of slightly cooled rice. Squeeze firmly, packing to make a round or triangle shape. Wrap the bottom with a quarter-cut piece of nori as seen in the image, covering the bottom evenly. Repeat until you run out of rice.

You can coat the outside of the rice with furikake or gomashio. But traditionally, most onigiri is served straight up: rice, filling, wrapped in nori seaweed. Itadakimasu!

japanese rice cup versus U.S. cup

A Japanese rice cup is different from a U.S. measuring cup. The standard cup size in the U.S. is 8 ounces. The standard cup of rice in Japan is ⅔ U.S. cup (6 ounces).

When purchasing a Japanese rice cooker (which I recommend!), be sure to pay attention to the water and rice measurements. If you're measuring with a Japanese rice cup, stick to Japanese rice cup water measurements as well. If you're using a U.S. cup, stick to U.S. water measurements. This will ensure that you have perfectly cooked rice.

A general rule of thumb: For every Japanese cup of rice, use 1 cup of water. For every U.S. cup of rice, use 1¼ cups water.

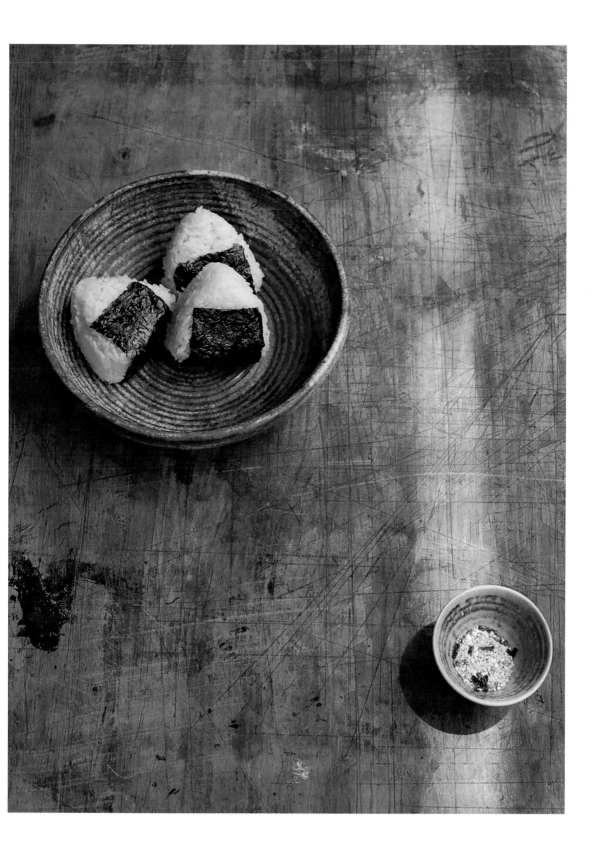

miso-carrot-cucumber salad

Serves 4 as an appetizer or side dish

This lightly seasoned salad was a favorite of mine growing up, close to a sunomono, a Japanese cucumber salad dish. I've added sweet, spiralized carrots here, and Mom likes to add extra fresh ginger to this refreshing summer side dish.

MISO DRESSING

2 tablespoons organic red or white miso paste

1 tablespoon toasted sesame oil

3 tablespoons rice vinegar or raw unfiltered apple cider vinegar

2 teaspoons toasted sesame seeds

SALAD

2 large cucumbers, julienned

1 large carrot, spiralized

2 tablespoons reconstituted wakame

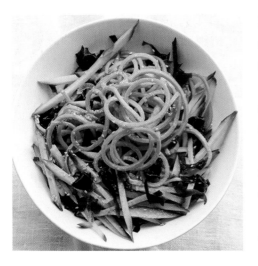

Make the dressing: Whisk together the miso paste, oil, vinegar, and toasted sesame seeds in a large bowl.

Assemble the salad: Add the sliced cucumbers, spiralized carrot, and wakame and toss to coat with the dressing.

Serve immediately, or make slightly in advance, cover, and refrigerate until chilled before serving, 10 to 20 minutes.

Leftovers can be stored in an airtight container in the fridge for up to 5 days.

avo nattō

Serves 4 as a snack

Nattō, beloved by the Japanese, is made of fermented soybeans. Nattō is definitely an acquired taste, and you may have to adjust to the very sticky texture as well as the smell, but I personally love the delicious fermented flavor of this Japanese delicacy. In this simple dish, the avocado mellows the pungency of the nattō.

4 cups cooked brown rice or your favorite grain

2 avocados, pitted, peeled, and cubed

Two 1.7-ounce packages organic nattō

TOPPINGS

Tamari soy sauce, low sodium or regular

Rice vinegar

Katsuobushi (Japanese dried bonito flakes; optional)

Scallions, thinly sliced on the bias

Divide the cooked brown rice or grains among four bowls.

Top off with the nattō and avocado cubes, followed by soy sauce, rice vinegar, and katsuobushi (if using), plus some thinly sliced scallions.

miso-roasted sweet potatoes

Serves 4

What happens when you add a touch of maple, sesame, rice vinegar, and miso to sweet, slow-roasted sweet potatoes? Heaven. For a quicker version of this recipe, go ahead and slice your favorite root veggies or sweet potatoes into 1-inch pieces/cubes, toss with a marinade, and roast on a baking sheet at 375°F for 40 minutes.

Nonstick olive or coconut oil cooking spray

3 tablespoons organic red or white miso paste

3 tablespoons toasted sesame oil

2 tablespoons rice vinegar

2 teaspoons organic maple syrup or honey

5 medium sweet potatoes or yams, peeled

Gomashio, for garnish

Preheat the oven to 400°F. Spray a nonstick 8- or 9-inch pie plate with cooking spray.

In a small bowl, combine the miso paste, sesame oil, vinegar, and maple syrup and whisk well to incorporate.

Neatly cut the potatoes into $1/4$-inch-thick chips on the bias. Line your sweet potatoes in the prepared pie plate and pour the marinade over them. Using a pastry brush, coat the sweet potatoes with the marinade. Cover with aluminum foil and allow the sweet potatoes to marinate at room temperature for about 30 minutes.

Place the foil-covered sweet potatoes on the bottom rack of the oven and roast for about 40 minutes, or until browned and tender.

Carefully remove the foil from the sweet potatoes and move the pan to the middle rack. Roast for 30 minutes more, uncovered. Watch carefully to prevent burning, and remove from the oven when the potatoes are tender and golden on the outside.

Serve the slightly cooled gorgeous roasted potatoes in their baking dish, family-style.

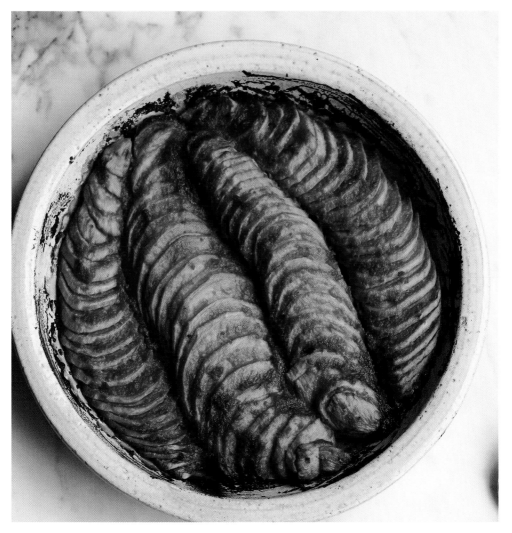

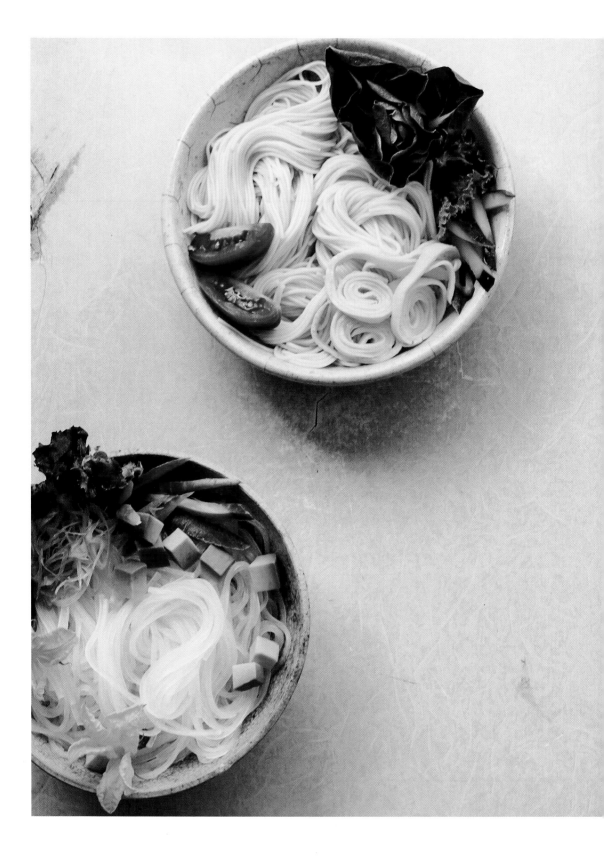

noodles
& soups

麺類，めんるい

スープ

menrui & shiru

easy miso soup with root veggies

Serves 4

Not into raw scallions? Swap in a handful of chopped leafy greens instead. Chard and kale, with their hearty textures, stand up well to the heat of the soup.

This delicious miso soup was inspired by my Baachan and her love of eating miso shiru every morning with gohan and tsukemono (Japanese pickles). When I make this simple, nourishing soup, I'm reminded of her daily rituals and motivated to create my own healthy habits.

4½ cups water

¼ cup organic red miso paste

¼ cup dried wakame

1 cup peeled and sliced root veggies (carrots, turnips, parsnips)

1 cup ¾-inch firm organic tofu (about half a 14-ounce package)

3 green onions, thinly sliced on the bias

Bring the water to a boil in a medium saucepan. Whisk in the miso and reduce the heat to low. When the liquid is at a simmer, add the dried wakame, followed by the veggies. Allow the soup to gently simmer for 6 to 7 minutes; do not boil.

Turn off the heat. Add the cubed tofu and allow to warm through, 1 to 2 minutes.

Ladle the soup into individual bowls and sprinkle with the green onions. Serve hot!

red potato + onion shiitake miso soup

Serves 6

This super-delicious and hearty soup is one of my favorites to make in the fall and winter months. With the addition of red potatoes, earthy shiitake mushrooms, and extra wakame, it's a truly satisfying meal.

3 tablespoons toasted sesame oil

1 yellow onion, thinly sliced

2½ cups thinly sliced shiitake mushroom caps

½ cup organic red or white miso paste (reduced sodium works, too)

2 tablespoons mirin

8 cups purified water

4 to 5 medium red potatoes, washed, patted dry, halved, and cut into 1-inch pieces

½ cup dried wakame

Shichimi tōgarashi spice or sriracha sauce, for those who like it hot! (optional)

Heat the oil in a large stockpot over medium-low heat. Add the sliced onion and sauté, stirring occasionally with a spatula, until light golden brown, about 12 minutes. Add the mushrooms and sauté until golden, 6 to 8 minutes more.

Add the miso paste. Mix well to combine and coat the onion and mushrooms with the paste. Sauté for an additional 5 minutes. Add the mirin and deglaze the pan.

Pour in the purified water and stir well to dissolve the miso paste. Increase the heat to medium-high and bring the mixture to a simmer. Add the potatoes, cover the pot, and let the soup cook for about 10 minutes, or until the potatoes can be pierced with a knife. Add the wakame and cook for about 5 minutes more. (If using long wakame strips, break them into small pieces over the pot.)

Ladle the soup into four serving bowls and top with tōgarashi, if desired.

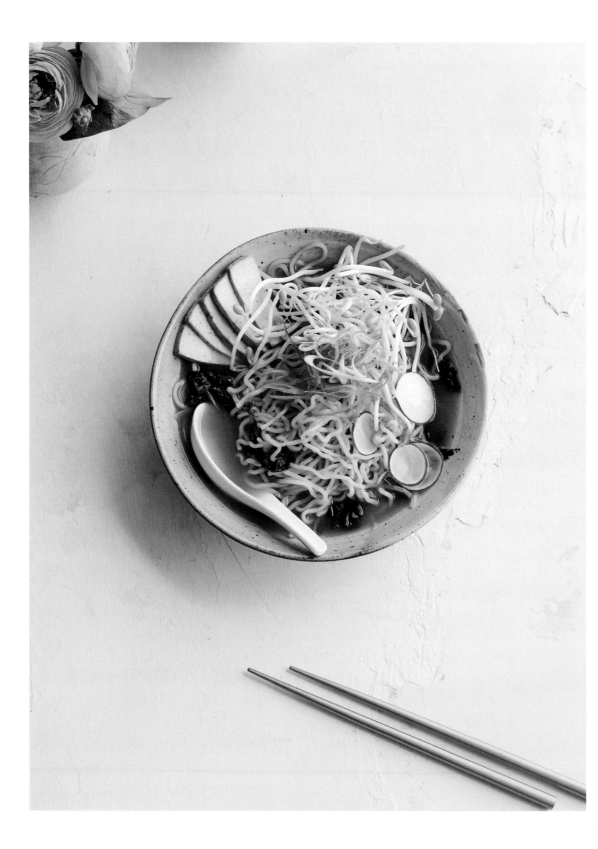

easy veggie ramen

Serves 2 or 3

Ramen—my absolute favorite Japanese meal. Mom raised us on this stuff. She and Dad would pack up the Volvo station wagon in San Diego, and drive us to L.A. once a month just to shop at the Japanese store in Gardena and get real Kyūshū ramen in Sherman Oaks. As the recipe title suggests, this one is super easy and packed with nutritious veggies. Every time I make it, I'm reminded of all those car rides, and nostalgic for the steaming bowls of ramen that resulted!

SOUP

2 tablespoons toasted sesame oil

1 small yellow onion, halved and thinly sliced

1 cup 1-inch cubes savory baked tofu (see page 162; optional)

2 cups thinly sliced collard or mustard greens

6 cups low-sodium vegetable broth or chicken stock

3 tablespoons reduced-sodium tamari soy sauce

One 10-ounce package fresh ramen noodles (Sun Noodle brand is the best) (If using dried approx. 3.55 ounces in size. Discard the seasoning packet.)

FRESH TOPPINGS

1 cup bean sprouts

1 green onion, thinly sliced on the bias

1 radish, thinly sliced (optional)

Chili oil or sriracha, for drizzling (the drizz!) (optional)

Tōgarashi (optional)

Toasted sesame seeds (optional)

Make the soup: In a medium pot over medium heat, combine the toasted sesame oil and onion and sauté for about 10 minutes, or until soft and translucent. Add the tofu (if using) and collard or mustard greens and sauté until the tofu has warmed through and the greens have wilted. Pour in the broth or stock along with the tamari. Increase the heat to a simmer. Cook just for a few minutes or until all the tofu and veggies are warmed through (do not overcook the greens).

Meanwhile, in a separate medium pot, add enough water to cook your noodles, and bring to a boil. Add the ramen noodles and cook for about 3 minutes, or as directed on the package. Remove from the heat and drain.

Taste the broth for seasoning, and add more tamari and/or a touch of mirin if needed, then turn the heat off.

Using tongs, divide the ramen noodles among individual serving bowls. Ladle the hot soup over the noodles and top with bean sprouts, green onions, and radish, if desired. Drizzle (the drizz!) with sriracha or chili oil and sprinkle with tōgarashi and/or toasted sesame seeds, if desired.

ramen notes

Ramen noodles are not meant to be served as "to-go" meals. Sure, ramen is meant to be quick, delicious, and simple, but never compromised. In fact, traditional ramen broth can take months to mature and perfect. The noodles must be consumed right after the broth is added, and perfecting the tare/soup base is a precise art.

Even in New York City, authentic ramen joints won't do takeout, which compromises the integrity of the noodle. Don't let this scare you away from trying my quickie recipe, but do steer clear of MSG-laden microwavable ramen.

When looking for ramen noodles, keep an eye out for my friend Kenshiro's ramen noodles, Sun Noodle brand. His fresh ramen noodles are handcrafted in the U.S. and Hawaii and the business is still owned and operated by his Japanese family. Their fresh noodles are *the best you can buy* for your homemade recipes. I highly recommend purchasing the *kaedama* noodles, as you can create your own flavorful broths with them! Trust me, I've tested them all, and have been using this family's brand for years, and I can't get enough!

nabe ryōri japanese hotpot (donabe)
土鍋 どなべ (nabemono) 鍋物, なべ物
kabocha squash daikon veggie nabe

Serves 4

Donabe means "hot pot" in Japanese. This beloved way of cooking a simple one-pot meal is as popular in Japan as the slow cooker is in the U.S. The Japanese love cooking nabe hot pots, especially in the cold winter months. My goal? To make this simple and delicious style of cooking much more popular in the U.S. Nabe pots are meant to be shared among a group, so gather a crowd and dig in!

3 tablespoons toasted sesame oil

1 yellow onion, thinly sliced into half-moons

2 cups thinly sliced shiitake mushroom caps

3 cups thinly sliced collard greens, kale leaves, or mizuna greens, stems reserved and finely chopped

1 tablespoon grated fresh ginger

7 tablespoons reduced-sodium organic red or white miso paste

2 tablespoons mirin

6 cups purified water

½ large daikon, peeled, halved lengthwise, and sliced thinly into half-moons

3 cups 1-inch cubes unpeeled kabocha squash

1 to 2 cups 1-inch cubes super-firm tofu

Tōgarashi, for sprinkling (optional)

In a large stockpot over medium-low heat, warm the oil. Add the onion and cook until translucent and fragrant, about 10 minutes.

Add the mushrooms and kale or collard stems and sauté until slightly golden, about 5 minutes. Add the grated ginger and cook until fragrant.

Add the miso paste, stir well to coat the onion and mushrooms with the paste, and cook for another 5 minutes. Deglaze the pan with the mirin. Add the water.

Neatly add the daikon slices, followed by the kabocha squash cubes. Increase the heat to medium-high, bring to a light simmer, and cook for about 8 minutes.

Add the tofu cubes. Add the thinly sliced greens and cook just to wilt.

To serve family-style, place a trivet or hot pad on your table and place the hot pot on top. Place a serving spoon with the pot and set out individual serving bowls. It is tradition to serve yourself, or have the host serve what veggies and protein you'd individually like from your nabe (try using chopsticks!) hot pot. Then ladle the hot broth on top of your veggies and tofu, and sprinkle with tōgarashi, if desired. Itadakimasu!

nabe hot pot love

nabe ryōri; 鍋料理 なべ りょうり hot pot cooking

donabe; 土鍋 どなべ clay pot

nabemono; 鍋物 なべもの food cooked in a hot pot, "nabe" shortened version

You can also pour the donabe broth over cooked rice and eat!

You can add leftover rice to your nabe pot and make porridge, aka Japanese okayu.

If you want to add any more flavors to your nabe pot, simply add salt, soy sauce (shōyu), or more miso paste.

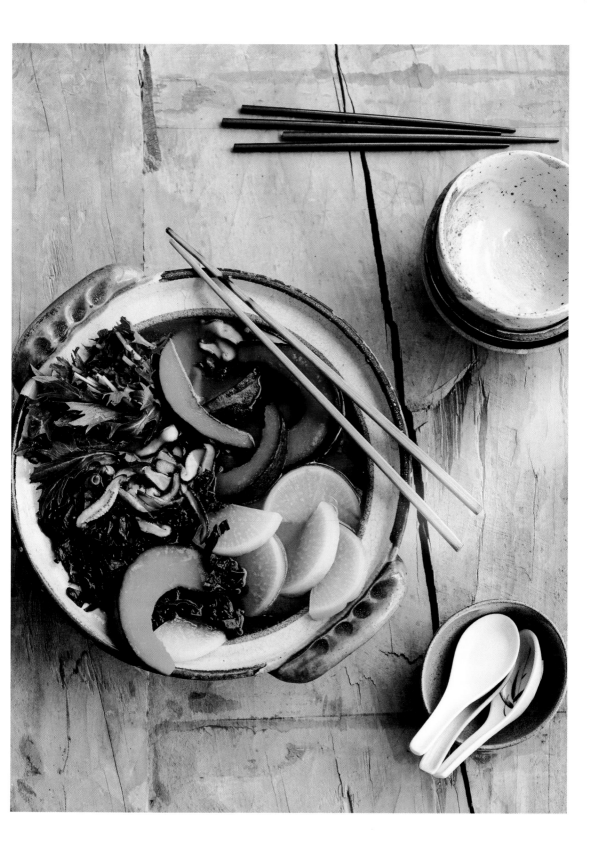

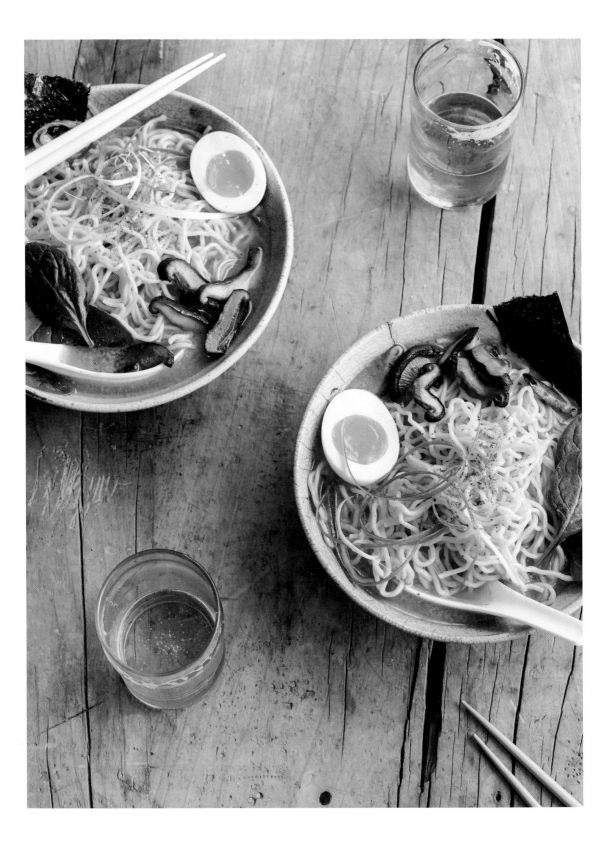

spicy miso-tahini ramen

Serves 4

This super-oishii ("delicious") spicy ramen bowl is made with basic pantry staples, such as miso paste and tahini, plus sriracha for spice! I love adding a bit more sriracha for heat, and topping it all off with a slightly runny soft-boiled egg.

SOUP

2 tablespoons toasted sesame oil

1 yellow onion, thinly sliced

2 cups thinly sliced shiitake mushroom caps

½ cup organic red miso paste

¼ cup tahini paste or neri goma (see sidebar)

2 tablespoons mirin

8 cups purified water

2 tablespoons Japanese chili paste or sriracha sauce

Two 10-ounce packages fresh ramen noodles (look for Sun Noodle brand, and check ounces to ensure the proper amount of noodles)

FRESH TOPPINGS

2 cups baby spinach

2 green onions, thinly sliced on the bias

2 soft-boiled eggs, sliced in half (optional)

1 avocado, pitted, peeled, and thinly sliced

Chili oil, for drizzling (optional)

Tōgarashi, for sprinkling (optional)

Nori, cut into small rectangular pieces, for dipping (optional)

Make the soup: In a large saucepan or stockpot, warm the toasted sesame oil over medium heat. Add the onion and sauté for 8 to 10 minutes, or until fragrant and translucent. Add 1 cup of the mushrooms and sauté for 2 to 3 minutes more.

Add the miso paste and tahini and stir to coat the onion and mushrooms. Cook for another 2 to 3 minutes. Watch your heat carefully and reduce to medium-low, if needed, or the soup can "break" or separate. Pour in the mirin and deglaze the pan. Pour in the water and stir well to dissolve all the miso paste.

Bring the soup up to a light simmer over high heat and whisk in the chili paste or sriracha sauce; start with 2 tablespoons to be safe, then add more as desired, and mix well to dissolve. Reduce the heat to medium-high.

In a separate medium saucepan, bring some water to a boil. Add the ramen noodles, and cook for 3 to 4 minutes. Using tongs, remove the noodles from the boiling water or drain the noodles in a colander.

Divide the noodles among four bowls. Add the spinach and green onions to each bowl. Top each bowl equally with the reserved 1 cup mushrooms, the egg, avocado, chili oil, tōgarashi, and nori as desired, ladle broth over, and serve.

tahini and neri goma

Tahini is a lightly roasted sesame seed paste, and is one of my favorite ingredients to cook with. *Neri goma* is Japanese roasted sesame seed paste, made with black and/or white unhulled or hulled sesame seeds. In Japan, it's standard to use neri goma. In the U.S., tahini is much more popular. And while the flavors can slightly vary (due to the degree of roasting, hulled or unhulled processing), I love cooking with both versions.

cali-style udon

Serves 4

Growing up, udon was a staple dish in our household. Mom was always crafting up delicious homemade dashi broth and throwing in all kinds of fresh local veggies. Topping my noodles off with greens, kabocha, avocados, and of course some furikake or gomashio is still my favorite way to enjoy udon. I prefer to cook with the thick udon noodles (fresh or frozen) versus dried, because this is the way mom did it.

DASHI

8 cups purified water

4 pieces kombu

1 cup katsuobushi (Japanese dried bonito flakes)

UDON SOUP

2 tablespoons toasted sesame oil

½ yellow onion, thinly sliced

2 cups bunashimeji mushrooms (bottoms removed) or thinly sliced shiitake mushroom caps

2 tablespoons mirin

1 teaspoon organic sugar

¼ cup reduced-sodium tamari soy sauce

Three 8-ounce packages frozen udon noodles, or 8 to 10 ounces dried udon noodles

TOPPINGS

1 cup fresh white corn kernels, shaved from about 2 ears

4 thin slices kamaboko (love the pink!), (optional)

1 ripe avocado, pitted, peeled, and thinly sliced

½ sheet nori, cut into small strips

1 cup arugula or baby spinach

1 tablespoon black gomashio

Tōgarashi

2 hard-boiled eggs, halved (optional)

Prepare the homemade dashi: In a medium saucepan over medium-high heat, bring the water and kombu pieces to a boil. Reduce the heat to medium-low and continue to simmer for 30 minutes. Turn off the heat. Add the katsuobushi and set aside until infused, 5 to 10 minutes longer. Strain the flavored broth, and reserve the liquid. You've got dashi!

Make the udon soup: In a separate medium to large stockpot, warm the oil over medium-high heat. Add the thinly sliced onion and sauté until fragrant, 8 to 10 minutes. Add the mushrooms and sauté for 4 to 5 minutes more.

Reduce the heat to medium. Add the mirin and deglaze the pan, then continue to cook, stirring, to evaporate all the liquid. Reduce the heat to medium-low and add the sugar and tamari soy sauce.

Carefully pour in the homemade dashi, bring to a light simmer, and cook for about 10 minutes.

In a separate pot, bring some water to a boil, add the udon noodles, and cook for 1 to 2 minutes, or as directed on the package. Remove from the heat, and drain in a colander under cold running water to cool.

To serve, divide the noodles among four bowls and ladle in the soup. Top with freshly shaved corn, a slice of kamaboko (if using), avocado slices, nori, arugula or spinach, and gomashio. Sprinkle with tōgarashi and add an egg half, if desired. Itadakimasu!

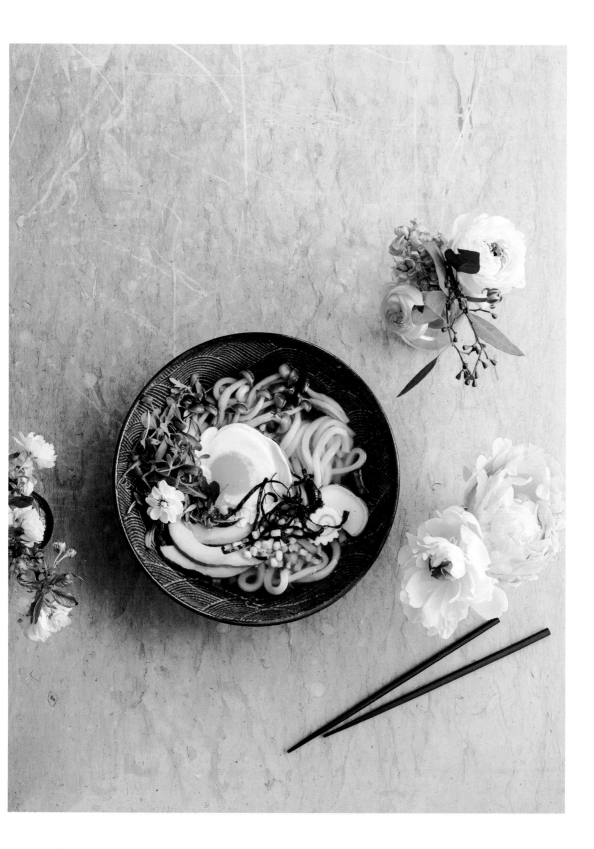

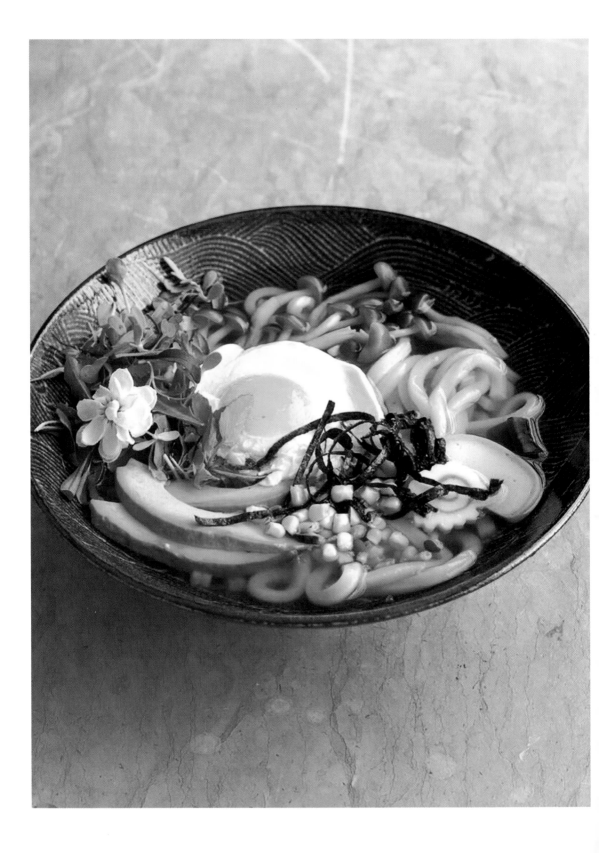

homemade dashi

Dashi is a basic soup stock used in Japanese cooking. You'll often hear chefs speak of "dashi" of all kinds—I was once served a strawberry dashi on Iron Chef America. *Fancy, right?*

Dashi in Japan is savory and, generally speaking, is made from three ingredients: katsuobushi (dried, fermented, thinly shaved bonito) and kombu (Japanese seaweed), plus water. The kombu is gently simmered in water, then the katsuobushi is added to infuse the umami flavor. The katsuobushi and kombu are removed and the hot liquid remaining is dashi! Different varieties can be made, too, like just kombu dashi or sometimes it's made with iriko *(small dried fish), sometimes with dried shiitake mushrooms, etc.*

This recipe makes a simple, clean, and basic dashi. You can use it in recipes throughout the book that call for dashi.

8 cups purified water

4 pieces kombu

1 cup katsuobushi (Japanese dried bonito flakes)

In a medium saucepan over medium-high heat, bring the kombu pieces and water to a boil. Reduce the heat to medium-low and simmer for 30 minutes.

Add the katsuobushi and simmer until the broth is infused, about 10 minutes more. Strain the flavored broth, and you've got dashi. Use immediately or store in an airtight jar in the fridge for up to 2 weeks.

summertime sōmen noodles

Serves 4

I love a bowl of cold noodles on a hot summer day. Try this simple one-pot dish for your next warm-weather meal.

NOODLES

One 9.5-ounce package sōmen noodles | 1 large bowl filled with 1 to 2 cups ice and water

OPTIONAL TOPPINGS (MIX AND MATCH AS YOU WISH)

Rice vinegar

Reduced-sodium tamari soy sauce

Sriracha sauce

Katsuobushi (Japanese dried bonito flakes)

Negi (green onions, thinly sliced on the bias)

Furikake (Japanese seaweed seasoning)

Arugula or your favorite leafy greens

Kaiware sprouts (daikon radish sprouts)

Gomashio (toasted, salted, crushed sesame seeds)

Tofu cubes

Avocado slices

In a large pot of boiling water, cook the sōmen noodles as directed on the package. Drain the noodles and place them in a large bowl filled with ice and water to serve. Your sōmen noodles will be the highlight of the table, so serve them up in a gorgeous bowl.

Serve family-style in the middle of your table. Using tongs or chopsticks, place the noodles into individual bowls, shaking off any residual water before serving.

Add your choice of sauces and toppings. I usually top with a touch of shōyu and rice vinegar, and offer a variety of toppings—negi, katsuobushi, arugula, tofu, avocado slices, etc.

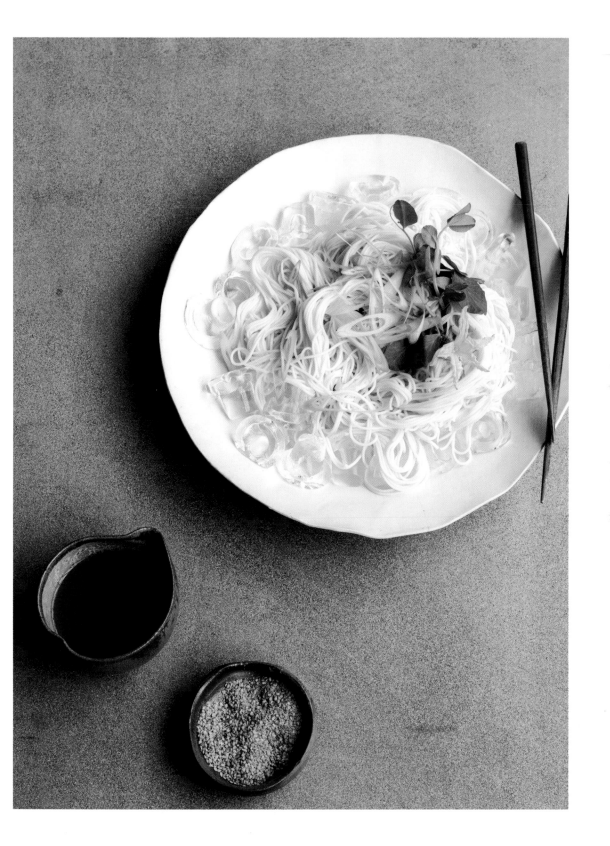

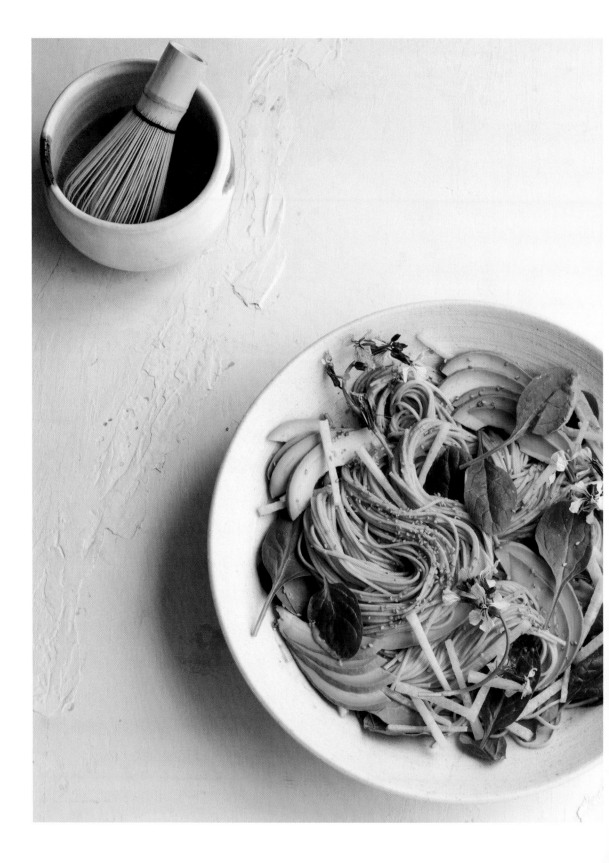

mains

メインコース

meinkōsu

sweet potato pancakes

Serves 4; makes about 12 pancakes

Inspired by my time in Okinawa, these pancakes are quite possibly the most perfect morning meal. With sweet potato puree, cinnamon, almond milk, and a touch of sea salt, they are a totally yum marriage of East meets West on a chilly fall morning.

2 cups all-purpose flour (gluten-free flour works, too!)

2 teaspoons aluminum-free baking powder

1½ teaspoons ground cinnamon

½ teaspoon sea salt

1½ cups sweet potato puree (or pumpkin puree if you'd like)

3 tablespoons organic sugar

3 large eggs

1 cup unsweetened almond milk

Coconut oil cooking spray

OPTIONAL TOPPINGS

Kinako powder (page 181)

Banana slices

Pure maple syrup

In a large bowl, whisk together the flour, baking powder, cinnamon, and salt.

In a medium bowl, whisk together the sweet potato puree, sugar, eggs, and almond milk. Slowly mix the wet ingredients into the dry ingredients; the batter will be thick.

Preheat a large nonstick skillet over medium heat. Coat the pan with nonstick cooking spray.

Using ⅓ cup of batter for each pancake, cook until the outer edges firm up and the bottom is golden brown, about 2 minutes. Flip and cook the other side until golden brown, about 2 more minutes.

Transfer the pancakes to a rimmed baking sheet and set aside. (You can keep them warm in the oven while you cook the rest, or serve them hot as you go!)

Continue cooking the remaining batter, transferring the pancakes to a plate or baking sheet as they are finished. To serve, plate up with your choice of kinako powder, banana slices, or maple syrup.

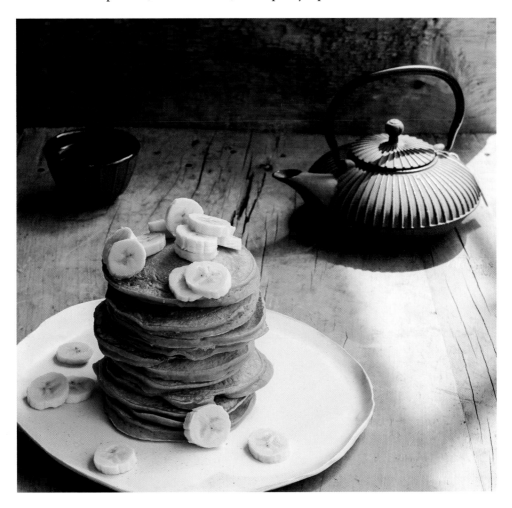

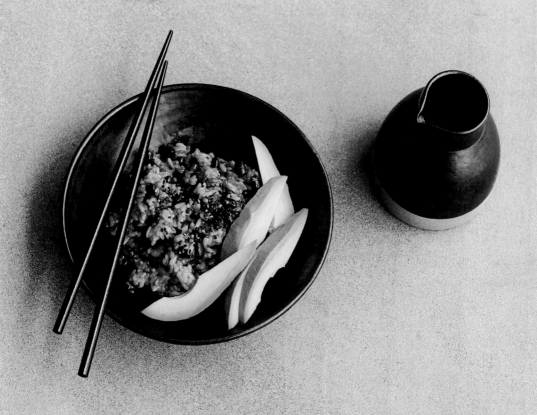
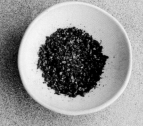

sekihan: traditional red bean rice
赤飯, せきはん

Serves 8 as a side dish

Sekihan is my favorite celebratory Japanese dish. Made of part sticky rice, part white rice, and red adzuki beans, this treat is typically made for celebrations like birthdays, weddings, anniversaries, and graduations. Some believe that you can consume sekihan for good luck. There are many ways to make sekihan, but I've found this balance of sticky mochigome (sweet mochi rice) and Japanese white rice to be a perfect blend.

1 cup dried red adzuki beans

1 cup white rice

2 cups mochi (sweet/sticky) rice (mochigome)

¾ teaspoon sea salt

1 tablespoon gomashio

STOVETOP OR RICE COOKER WATER MEASUREMENTS

If cooking rice on the stovetop: Combine rice with 2½ cups water and gently simmer over a medium-low heat, covered, for 20 to 25 minutes.

If using a rice cooker: Follow your rice cooker's instructions, measure to the 5-cup line, and cook for 45 minutes; a medium or large rice cooker is best. (See more on page 94.)

In a small colander or strainer, rinse the adzuki beans well and then drain. Put the adzuki beans in a medium or large pot along with 3 ½ cups water and bring to a boil.

Reduce the heat to medium-low and cook for 20 to 25 minutes.

After 25 minutes, the beans will be just about three-quarters of the way cooked. Turn off the heat. Remove the pot from the heat, place the lid on the pot, and allow both the beans and the cooking liquid to cool to room temperature.

In a medium bowl, wash, rinse, and drain both your white and sweet mochi rice thoroughly (see sidebar below).

Combine both types of rice in a large pot or rice cooker and gently add the cooked adzuki beans with their reserved liquid. Add the sea salt.

Give the mixture a quick stir to combine well and evenly distribute the salt, liquid, and beans.

When the rice is perfectly cooked, portion it into individual bowls, top with the gomashio, serve, and enjoy! Note that mochi rice is extra filling and this recipe is truly one of the most comforting parts of my childhood.

Save your leftovers for super-yummy sekihan onigiri (page 127).

PS: I lov-v-v-e this rice topped with a little tamari shōyu (soy sauce) and avocado slices!

washing rice

My mom always taught me to wash my rice prior to cooking. Washing your rice not only cleans it of dirt and grittiness, but also releases excess starch, thus preparing your rice for precise results. To wash your rice, simply place it in a large bowl or your rice cooker bowl. Pour cold water into your bowl, just enough to cover the rice. Agitate the rice using your clean hands. You'll notice the water will become slightly cloudy; this is the starch being washed off. Rinse with cool water, and carefully drain all the water from the rice. Repeat this process once more.

sekihan onigiri 赤飯お握り,せきはんおにぎり

Yields will vary depending on how much leftover rice you have

This recipe seriously makes me smile and feel like a kid again. Sekihan onigiri is a simple way to make a to-go lunch and it's made with your delish leftover sekihan rice. Mom recommends making a small onigiri (like **nigirizushi** 握り寿司, *the traditional oval sushi with fish on top) and wrapping it with a thin strip of nori.*

Sea salt

Leftover sekihan rice (see page 125)

Nori squares or strips

Fill a large bowl with ¹/₃ cup lukewarm water and a pinch of salt. Using this water, wet your clean hands.

Using your leftover sekihan rice, scoop about ¹/₃ cup of the cooled rice into your palm and mold it into a triangle shape, disk, or ball. Press firmly to pack the rice. Add nori strips to wrap if desired.

Continue to make onigiri until you run out of rice!

Eat immediately or wrap in plastic wrap or store in a reusable container and use parchment paper to separate the onigiri. Enjoy with a touch of shōyu!

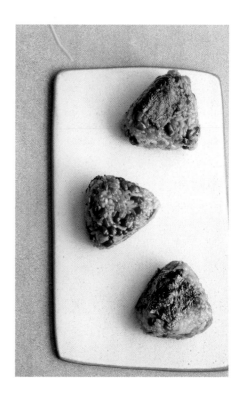

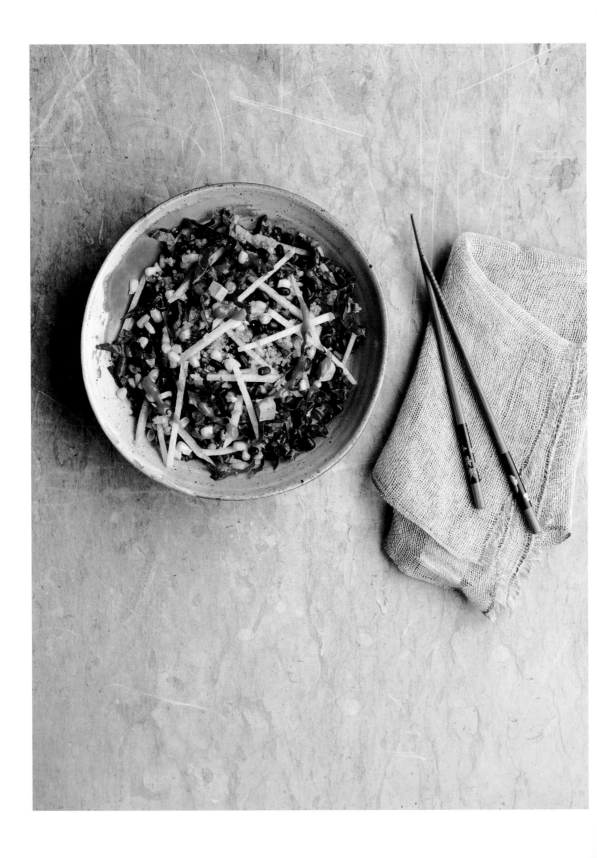

spicy miso, ginger, jicama, corn + kale chopped salad

Serves 2 as main meal

This super clean salad is so refreshing—I love the fresh crisp jicama mixed with the avocado, corn, and adzuki beans. Protein-rich and satisfying, it's a perfect post-workout or midday meal to get you through your afternoon.

MISO-GINGER VINAIGRETTE

3 tablespoons organic miso paste

1 teaspoon grated fresh ginger

½ teaspoon honey or pure maple syrup

3 tablespoons rice vinegar

2 tablespoons toasted sesame oil

1 to 2 tablespoons sriracha sauce

SALAD

1 bunch kale, stems removed, leaves chopped and massaged (simply wash, pat dry, chop, and with clean hands, delicately massage chopped leaves to slightly wilt)

1 cup cooled cooked quinoa (about ⅓ cup uncooked)

Kernels shaved from 1 ear fresh white corn

½ cup cooked adzuki beans

1 large jicama or daikon, sliced into matchsticks

1 avocado, pitted, peeled, and cubed

Savory baked tofu (page 162), if desired

In a large bowl, add the ingredients for the vinaigrette and whisk well to combine.

Toss in the kale and coat gently with the dressing. Once coated, add the rest of your ingredients and toss gently.

Add firm, savory tofu, if desired, and serve immediately.

miso kale caesar salad

Serves 2 as a main or 4 as small side salads

This salad is most definitely going to change the way you look at your basic Caesar salad. With tahini, miso, a touch of sweetness, and rice vinegar, this umami-lover's dream salad is the perfect way to put a fresh spin on a Western classic.

MISO CAESAR DRESSING

¼ cup tahini paste

¼ cup organic red or white miso paste

¼ cup rice vinegar

1 teaspoon honey or pure maple syrup

SALAD

1 large bunch lacinato or curly kale, stemmed, leaves finely chopped and massaged well (using clean hands, massage kale for 5 minutes to slightly wilt)

Kernels shaved from 1 ear raw white corn (about ½ cup kernels)

½ daikon radish, peeled, halved, and thinly sliced into half-moons (about 2 cups)

2 avocados, pitted, peeled, and cut into ¾-inch cubes

2 tablespoons gomashio or hemp seeds

Furikake or nori seaweed (optional)

In a medium bowl, whisk together all the ingredients for the dressing until well combined. Add the finely chopped lacinato kale, raw white corn, and daikon radish and toss well to combine with the dressing.

To serve, plate up your salad into serving bowls and top with cubed avocado, toasted sesame seeds or hemp seeds, and furikake or nori, if desired.

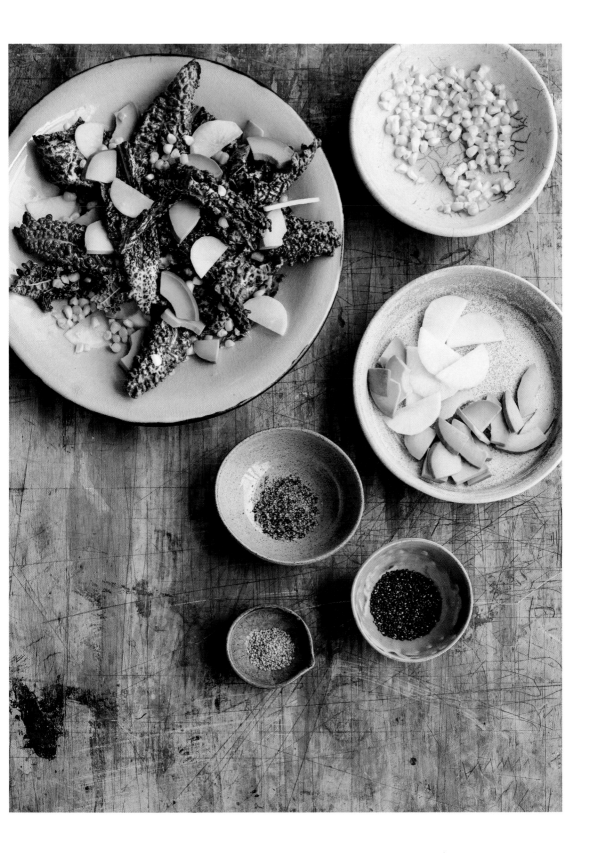

turmeric-kale fried rice

Serves 4

Mom always made a simple fried rice dish for us, particularly when she had leftover white rice, and I watched her create this oishii, one-pan meal using only leftovers! The simple addition of turmeric (or curry powder) instantly transforms plain old rice into a completely different dish.

2 cups uncooked brown rice (or your choice of grains)

2 tablespoons toasted sesame oil

½ large yellow onion, finely chopped

2 garlic cloves, finely minced

2 carrots, finely chopped

3 tablespoons reduced-sodium tamari soy sauce

3 green onions, finely sliced on the bias

1 tablespoon ground turmeric

1 cup ¾-inch cubes savory tofu

1 cup chopped kale or broccoli rabe

Gomashio, for topping (optional)

In a medium saucepan, bring brown rice, or your choice of grain, plus the appropriate amount of water to a boil. Reduce to a simmer and cook for 25 to 30 minutes until tender. Drain any excess liquid, fluff with a fork, and set aside to cool.

In medium sauté pan, heat the oil over medium heat. Add the yellow onion and sauté for about 8 minutes, or until translucent. Add the garlic and cook until fragrant. Add the carrots and cook approximately 2 minutes. Pour in the soy sauce and cook, stirring occasionally, until it begins to evaporate, about 2 minutes.

Add half the green onions and stir-fry for another 3 minutes, or until thoroughly heated. Sprinkle in the turmeric. Add the cooked rice or grains and sauté until warmed through. Add the tofu and warm through. Add the finely chopped kale or broccoli rabe and stir to coat and quickly warm through. Top with the remaining green onions, sprinkle with some go-mashio, if desired, and serve immediately.

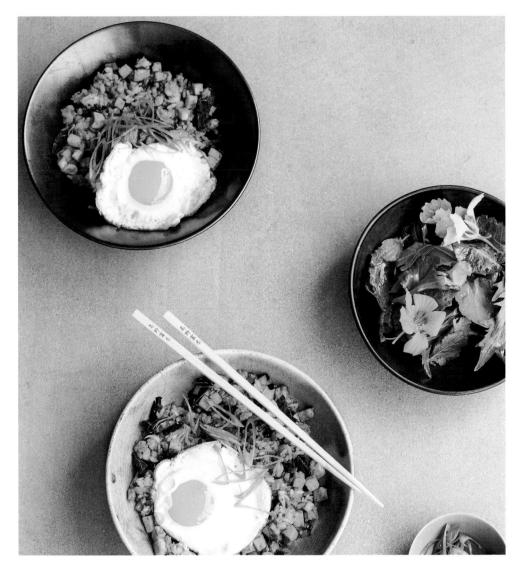

light yakisoba noodles
焼きそば, やきそば

Serves 3

Mom used to make this dish as a quick, filling meal for the family on busy days. Yakisoba is a simple, flavorful stir-fry noodle. Feel free to toss in your own leftover proteins and veggies to mix it up and make it your own!

2 tablespoons toasted sesame oil

½ yellow onion, finely diced

2 garlic cloves, minced

2 cups thinly sliced shiitake mushroom caps

3 cups fresh yakisoba noodles (look for these at the Japanese market)

2 cups finely chopped kale

1½ teaspoons toasted sesame seeds

LIGHT YAKISOBA SAUCE

2 tablespoons reduced-sodium tamari soy sauce

3 tablespoons rice vinegar

1 tablespoon tomato paste (or try sriracha!!)

¼ cup vegan Worcestershire sauce

¼ cup purified water

In a medium sauté pan warm the oil over medium heat. Add the onion and sauté for 5 minutes, stirring occasionally. Add the garlic and sauté for 2 minutes, until fragrant. Add the mushrooms and sauté for 2 to 3 minutes more, stirring well.

Add all the ingredients for the light yakisoba sauce to the pan and stir. Add the fresh yakisoba noodles and sauté for a few minutes, tossing to coat all the noodles with the sauce, and cook until the water evaporates.

Add the chopped kale and toss to slightly wilt and coat with the sauce. Divide the noodles among individual serving bowls and top with ½ teaspoon of sesame seeds per bowl.

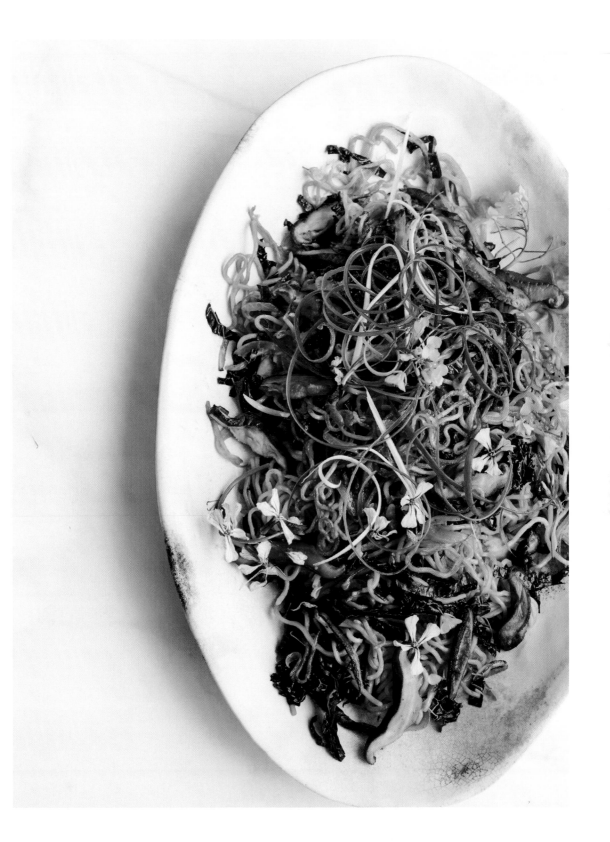

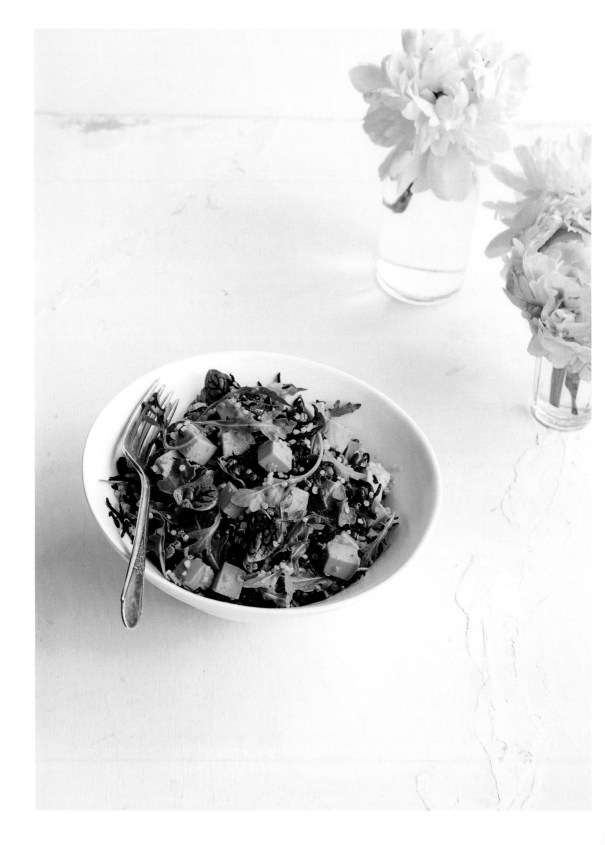

hijiki + avocado greens salad

Serves 2 as a full meal bowl, 3 or 4 as a side dish

This fresh, filling bowl is one of my favorite recipes in this book! If you're new to hijiki seaweed, this is a great entry-level dish to try. This super-simple and clean dressing contains only three ingredients, so you have no excuse not to make it yourself. This salad keeps well overnight in the fridge—so make a bowlful the night before and pack it for your lunch the next day!

1¼ cups plus 1 tablespoon dried hijiki seaweed

¾ cup water

3 cups cooked quinoa

One 15-ounce can adzuki beans, rinsed and drained

2 cups packed arugula or finely chopped kale

2 ripe avocados, pitted, peeled, and cut into ½-inch cubes

DRESSING

3 tablespoons reduced-sodium tamari soy sauce

¼ cup plus 2 tablespoons rice vinegar or raw unfiltered apple cider vinegar

2 tablespoons toasted sesame oil

In a medium bowl, soak and reconstitute the dried hijiki in the water for about 15 minutes. Drain the excess liquid.

In a large bowl, whisk together the soy sauce, vinegar, and oil. Add the reconstituted hijiki, quinoa, adzuki beans, and arugula to the dressing and toss to coat. Top with the avocado cubes and serve immediately at room temperature.

spicy tahini + avocado soba

Serves 4

Soba + tahini + avocado? Enough said. This full-meal noodle salad is one of my favorite ways to fill up on good carbs, healthy fats, and plenty of nutrient-rich greens.

TAHINI-MISO DRESSING

¼ cup tahini paste

3½ tablespoons organic red miso paste

¼ cup plus 1 tablespoon rice vinegar

1 to 2 tablespoons sriracha sauce (depending on how hot you like it)

NOODLE SALAD

One 8 to 9.5 ounce pack dried soba noodles

1 cup thin jicama matchsticks

2 cups baby spinach

1 avocado, pitted, peeled, and sliced

2 tablespoons gomashio, plus more as needed

In a medium saucepan, cook the soba noodles in boiling water, as directed on your package.

Make the dressing: Put the tahini paste, miso paste, rice vinegar, and sriracha in a large bowl. Whisk well.

Drain the cooked noodles and rinse under cold running water; set aside in the colander. (Quick tip: To keep your noodles from clumping together, rub the noodles together when rinsing under cold running water to wash away excess starch. This will also make sure your noodles maintain a perfect texture.)

Add your drained and cooled soba noodles to the dressing bowl and toss.

Add the jicama and baby spinach; mix well. Top off the soba noodles with avocado slices and gomashio.

To serve, twirl the noodles using tongs and place in individual bowls.

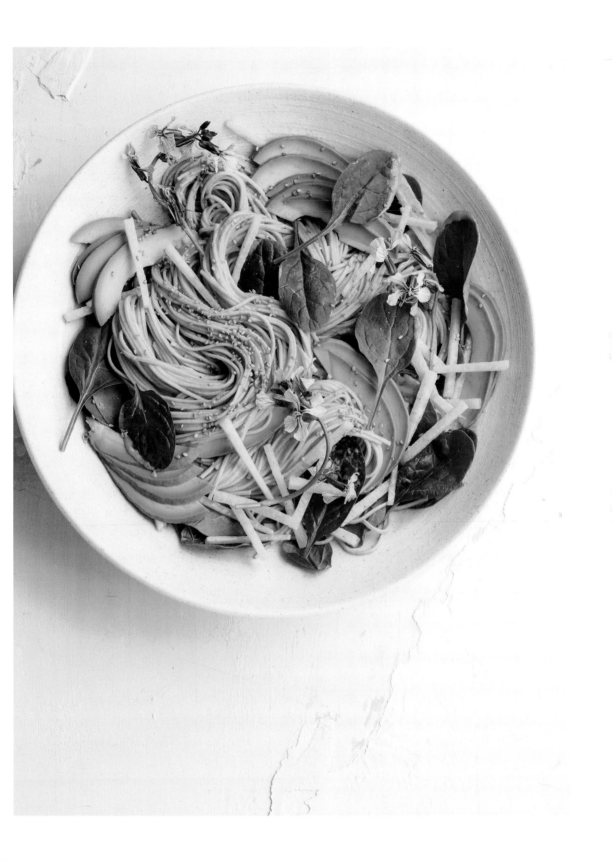

kale avocado soba bentō box

Serves 4

Bentō is one of my favorite Japanese food novelties, and these little lunchboxes are a super-delicious and fun way to get kids excited about healthy eating. Traditional bentō can be found all over Japanese department stores as well as train stations. Mom and I are completely obsessed with grabbing bentō as soon as we arrive in Nippon!

2 tablespoons toasted sesame oil

2 cups thinly sliced shiitake mushroom caps

1 tablespoon reduced-sodium tamari soy sauce

6 to 10 ounces soba noodles

4 cups chopped kale

1 cup organic edamame, cooked and shelled

1 avocado, peeled, pitted, and thinly sliced

2 cups arugula

1 to 2 teaspoons toasted sesame seeds

MISO-GINGER DRESSING

3 tablespoons organic red miso paste

⅓ cup rice vinegar or raw unfiltered apple cider vinegar

2 tablespoons toasted sesame oil

1 tablespoon grated fresh ginger, or 1 teaspoon ground ginger

2 teaspoons honey or pure maple syrup

In a large sauté pan, warm the oil over medium heat. Add the mushrooms and cook until fragrant, approximately 6 minutes. Add the soy sauce and cook just until evaporated. Set the mushrooms aside.

In a medium saucepan, cook the soba noodles as directed on the package. Drain and rinse the noodles under cold running water and set aside.

Make the dressing: In a large bowl, whisk together the miso paste, vinegar, oil, ginger, and honey.

Add the kale to the bowl and toss to coat well with the dressing. Add the drained soba noodles, edamame, and mushrooms and gently toss again until everything is well coated in the dressing. Top with the avocado slices, arugula, and sesame seeds. Have fun and get creative plating up your bentō box!

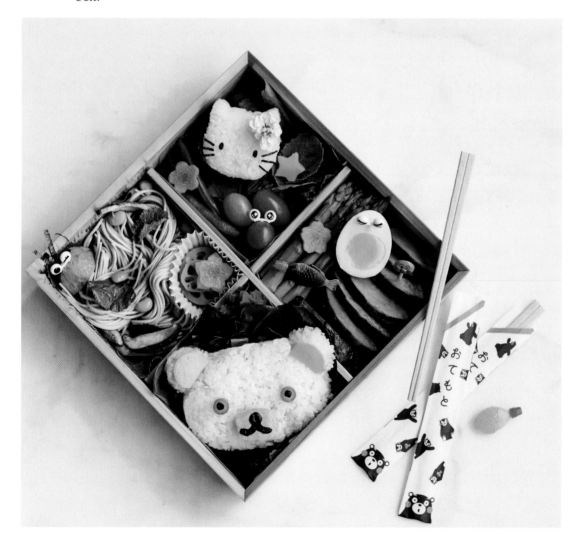

roasted miso sweet potato + kale salad

Serves 2

This hearty and delicious salad is made with miso-roasted potatoes and kale, protein-packed quinoa, and crunchy cucumbers. I love this delicate orange miso dressing, which complements the flavors of the sweet potatoes so beautifully. This is one recipe you'll keep coming back to for a simple, hassle-free dinner bowl!

SALAD

Approximately ½ cup uncooked quinoa

1 bunch kale, finely chopped

1 small Persian cucumber or Japanese kyūri, cut into thin half-moons

SWEET POTATOES

Coconut oil cooking spray

2 large sweet potatoes or yams

2 tablespoons organic red miso paste

1 tablespoon mirin

2 tablespoons unrefined coconut oil, melted

Gomashio

ORANGE-MISO DRESSING

1 teaspoon finely grated orange zest

¼ cup freshly squeezed orange juice

1 tablespoon reduced-sodium tamari soy sauce

2 tablespoons organic white miso paste

2 tablespoons rice vinegar

2 tablespoons mirin

Make the sweet potatoes: Preheat the oven to 350°F. Line a baking sheet with parchment paper or aluminum foil and spray with cooking spray.

At the same time, in a medium saucepan, cook the quinoa until just slightly undercooked. Turn off the heat, set the quinoa aside.

Using a sharp knife, cut the sweet potatoes into 1-inch cubes (be sure not to cube them too small since they will shrink during roasting!).

Combine the cubed sweet potatoes, miso paste, mirin, and coconut oil on the prepared baking sheet and toss to coat.

Roast the sweet potatoes for 38 to 40 minutes, tossing halfway through the roasting time to ensure even cooking.

Meanwhile, make the dressing: In a large bowl, whisk together the dressing ingredients to combine.

Add the quinoa, chopped kale, and cucumbers and toss to coat well with the dressing.

Serve the quinoa and kale salad in your favorite serving bowl(s) or on a large platter, and top with the roasted sweet potatoes and gomashio. Itadakimasu!

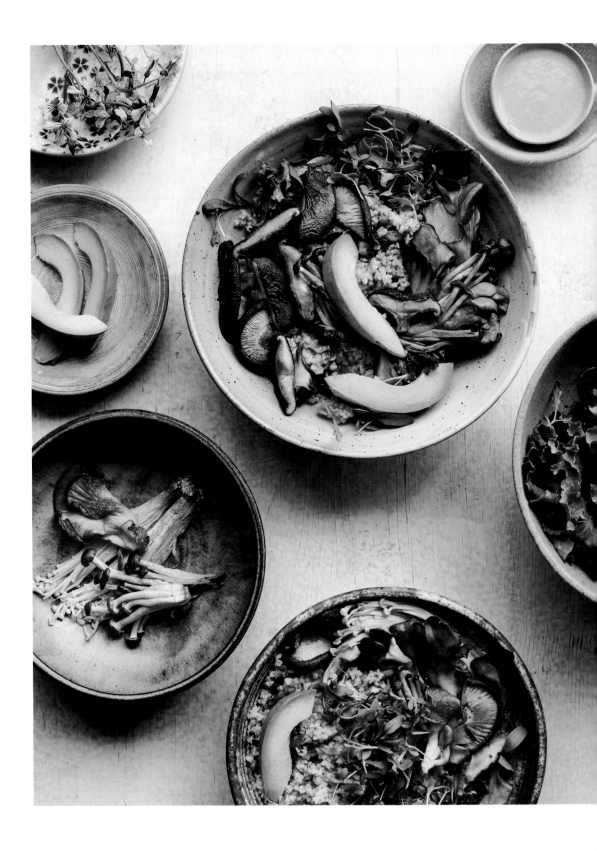

big bowls

丼，どんぶり

donburi

avocado-miso-mushroom bowl

Serves 2 as large bowls, or 4 as a side dish

I wrote this recipe as I was thinking about those fall and winter months when all I want is a quick, leftover grain—based meal to whip up and impress. This meal comes together quickly and is deeply satisfying. Of course, you can add your favorite choice of greens, grains, and any other toppings!

SALAD

- 2 tablespoons toasted sesame oil or extra-virgin olive oil
- 6 cups thinly sliced mixed mushrooms: shiitake, maitake, bunashimeji, or your fave mushrooms
- 1 tablespoon reduced-sodium tamari soy sauce
- 4 cups cooked grains: your choice of brown rice, freekeh, farro, or quinoa

- 1 tablespoon mirin
- 4 cups packed fresh greens, such as arugula or finely chopped kale leaves (reserve 3 cups for the salad, 1 cup for topping)
- 1 ripe avocado, pitted, peeled, and thinly sliced
- 2 teaspoons crushed gomashio, for topping

CREAMY MISO-TAHINI DRESSING

- 2 tablespoons organic miso paste
- 3 tablespoons tahini paste

- ¼ cup plus 2 tablespoons rice vinegar

In a large sauté pan, warm the sesame oil or extra-virgin olive oil over medium heat. Add the mushrooms and sauté until lightly golden, 3 to 4 minutes. Add the tamari and sauté for 2 minutes more. Deglaze the pan with the mirin to release the bits from the bottom of the pan. Turn off heat.

In a large bowl, whisk together the ingredients for the dressing. Using a spatula, stir in the grains and fully coat. Add the mushrooms and 3 cups of the greens, and gently fold to coat well with the dressing.

Top with the avocado, reserved greens, and gomashio.

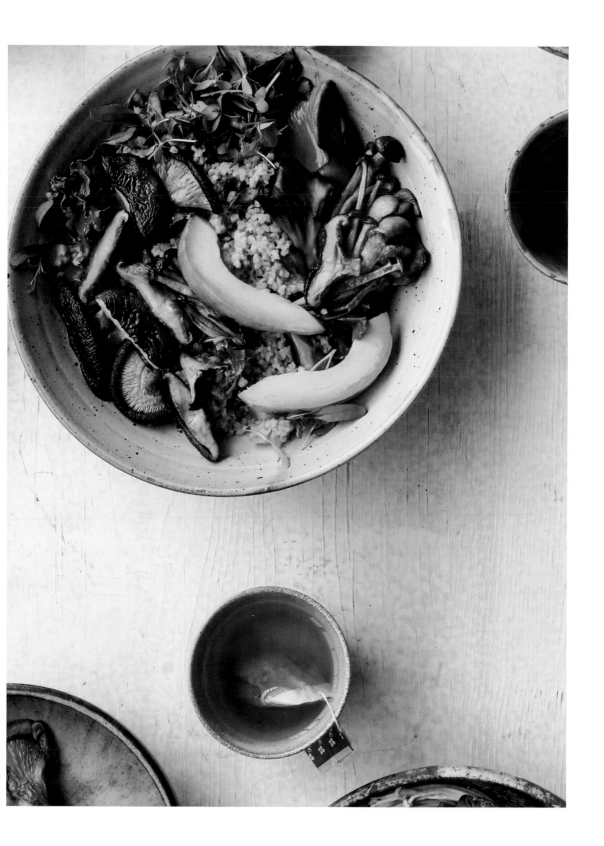

roasted kabocha bowl

Serves 4

If you haven't tried roasting kabocha squash yet, this is the perfect recipe. You'll love the richness of kabocha, which has a delicate pumpkin-like flavor. The tamari-ginger dressing also offers the perfect balance of salt, acid, sweet, and umami.

4 cups cubed skin-on kabocha squash

2 medium yams, unpeeled and cubed

4 tablespoons extra-virgin olive oil

2 cups cooked brown rice (leftovers are the best!)

2 cups arugula, chopped spinach, or kale

One 6-ounce package store-bought savory tofu, such as Wildwood brand, cut into ¾-inch cubes, or 6 ounces homemade Savory Tofu (page 162)

TAMARI-GINGER DRESSING

⅓ cup rice vinegar

2 tablespoons toasted sesame oil

2 tablespoons reduced-sodium tamari soy sauce

1 tablespoon grated fresh ginger

½ teaspoon honey or pure maple syrup

2 cups arugula, chopped spinach, or kale

Preheat the oven to 375°F. Line one large or two smaller baking sheets with aluminum foil.

Place the squash and yams on the baking sheet(s) and toss with the 2 tablespoons of extra-virgin olive oil. Transfer to the oven and roast the yams for 35 to 40 minutes and the squash for 40 to 45 minutes, carefully tossing halfway through the roasting time.

Remove from the oven.

Make the dressing: In a large bowl, whisk together the vinegar, toasted sesame oil, tamari soy sauce, ginger, and honey/maple.

Add the cooked brown rice, your favorite greens, the roasted squash cubes, and the yam cubes. Toss to lightly coat all the ingredients with the dressing.

Add the cubed tofu and toss gently.

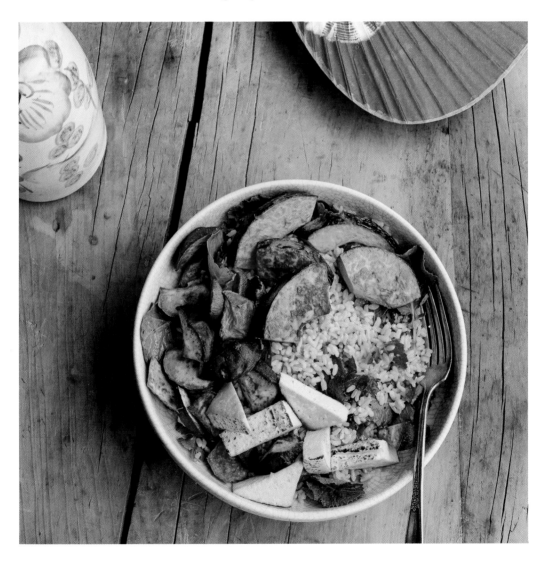

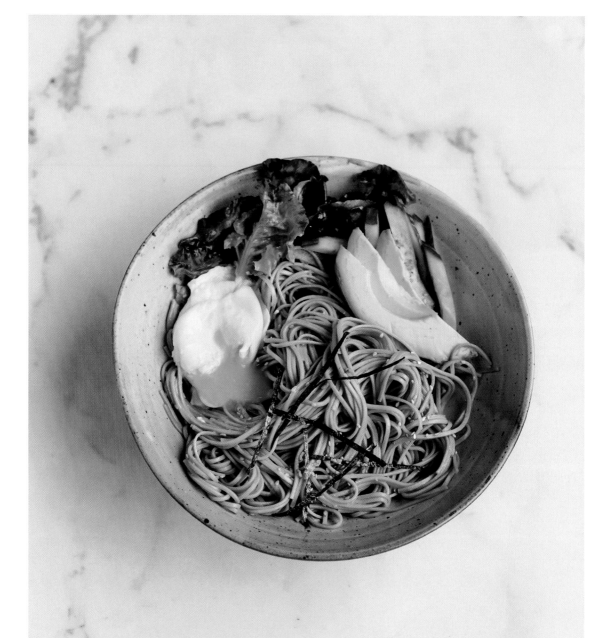

avocado soba greens bowl

Serves 3

Growing up with soba as a staple in our household, I remember Mom telling me and Sis that these buckwheat noodles would keep us strong. With the protein, prebiotics, and good carbs that soba noodles have to offer, they do make you feel nourished!

6 ounces soba noodles

½ cup thinly sliced cucumber half-moons

4 cups torn red-leaf lettuce

½ avocado, pitted, peeled, and thinly sliced

Toasted sesame seeds (garnish)

RED MISO-GINGER DRESSING

2 tablespoons organic red miso paste

⅓ cup rice vinegar or raw unfiltered apple cider vinegar

1 tablespoon toasted sesame seeds

2 teaspoons grated fresh ginger

1 teaspoon honey or pure maple syrup

Touch of toasted sesame oil (optional)

Poached egg, toasted nori strips (optional to top)

In a medium saucepan, bring water to a boil to cook your soba noodles according to the package directions. Drain and rinse the noodles in a colander under cold running water and set aside.

In a large bowl, whisk together the red miso paste, rice vinegar, toasted sesame seeds, ginger, honey, and a touch of toasted sesame oil, if desired. Add the drained soba noodles, sliced cucumber, and torn red-leaf lettuce. Gently toss until well coated in the dressing.

To serve, twirl the noodles using tongs, set them in individual serving bowls, and top with avocado slices and toasted sesame seeds, if desired.

hiyashi chūka 冷やし中華, ひやしちゅうか

Serves 4

Mom never ceases to amaze me. She's always got so many new recipes to share with me, and when I'm visiting back home in California, she goes all out to make me my favorite foods. One particularly hot summer day, she made hiyashi chūka *for me and Dad. Served as a cold noodle dish, it's light, simple, flavorful, and absolutely delicious. I enjoy it year-round; you will, too!*

8 to 9 ounces rice sōmen, fresh ramen, or Chinese yellow noodles (or try angel hair pasta!)

3 cups red-leaf lettuce, julienned

½ large cucumber, or 2 small, julienned (about 1¼ cups)

1 tomato, julienned (about ¾ cup)

1 avocado, pitted, peeled, and thinly sliced

1 green onion, thinly sliced on the bias, for garnish (optional)

Sesame seeds, for garnish (optional)

TAMAGOYAKI (JAPANESE OMELET)

1 teaspoon toasted sesame oil

2 large eggs, well beaten

1 tablespoon dashi or a touch of shōyu, if desired

HIYASHI CHŪKA SAUCE

¼ cup reduced-sodium tamari soy sauce

2 tablespoons toasted sesame oil

1 tablespoon toasted sesame seeds

1 teaspoon tōgarashi

2½ teaspoons grated fresh ginger

1 teaspoon honey or pure maple syrup

3 tablespoons rice vinegar

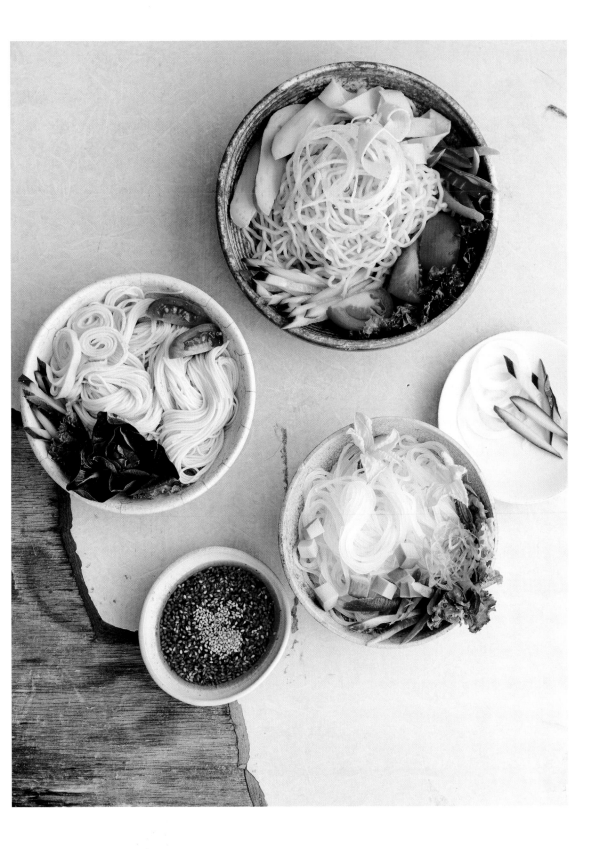

In a medium stockpot, bring a generous amount of water to a boil. Add the noodles and cook as directed on the package. Drain and rinse in a colander under cold running water and set aside.

Make the tamagoyaki: In a small nonstick pan, heat the sesame oil over medium-low heat. Pour in the beaten eggs and allow to set, 3 to 4 minutes. Once set, using chopsticks or a small spatula, fold the thin crepe-like eggs like you would a traditional omelet. Allow the tamagoyaki to cool for 1 to 2 minutes, then thinly slice it into strips.

Make the sauce: Add all the ingredients for the hiyashi chūka sauce to a large bowl and whisk well to combine. Add the noodles and lettuce and toss gently to coat with the dressing.

Using tongs, transfer the dressed noodles and lettuce to individual serving bowls and top with the sliced cucumber, tomato, tamagoyaki, and avocado. Add green onions and/or toasted sesame seeds as a garnish, if desired.

tamagoyaki

Just as in French cuisine, where there is not one single way to make a great omelet, every Japanese cook makes his or her tamagoyaki a little differently. Some cooks love adding dashi, sugar, or mirin; others add shōyu. I'd encourage you to experiment and find the combination you love best—there are no rules!

roasted carrot + avocado bowl with carrot-miso vinaigrette

Serves 4

After many years of testing and developing recipes, I found a new love for roasting carrots. I was never that excited about carrots before, but I find that with the addition of curry powder and coconut oil, they are absolutely irresistible. Combined with my other favorites—miso, avocado, and quinoa— they are even better!

GRAIN BOWL

- 2 tablespoons unrefined virgin coconut oil, melted
- 2 tablespoons organic red or white miso paste
- 2 teaspoons curry powder
- 6 carrots, cut into 1-inch pieces on the bias
- 6 cups cooked quinoa, brown rice, or farro (or your favorite grains)
- 1 ripe avocado, pitted, peeled, and cut into 1-inch cubes
- 2 cups finely chopped red-leaf lettuce
- 1 cup leftover roasted vegetables (optional)
- 2 tablespoons gomashio, for topping

MISO-CARROT VINAIGRETTE (makes about 1½ cups)

- 3 medium carrots, roughly chopped into ½-inch pieces
- 2 tablespoons roughly chopped yellow onion
- 3 tablespoons organic miso paste
- 2 tablespoons unrefined virgin coconut oil or extra-virgin olive oil
- 1 tablespoon toasted sesame oil
- ½ cup rice vinegar
- 2 tablespoons water

Preheat the oven to 375°F. Line a baking sheet with aluminum foil and coat with nonstick cooking spray.

In a medium bowl, whisk together the coconut oil, miso, and curry powder. Add the carrots to the bowl and toss to coat well. Transfer the curried carrots to the prepared baking sheet. Roast for about 25 minutes, or until fully cooked and slightly golden brown. Remove from the oven.

While the carrots cook, make the vinaigrette: Place all the vinaigrette ingredients into a blender and blend until smooth. Add more water as needed.

In each of four individual serving bowls, add 1½ cups of the quinoa. Top each with an equal amount of avocado cubes, roasted carrots, red-leaf lettuce, and leftover roasted veggies, if using. Drizzle with 2 tablespoons of the vinaigrette, or more if you'd like. Top off with gomashio. Serve at room temperature, or heat if desired.

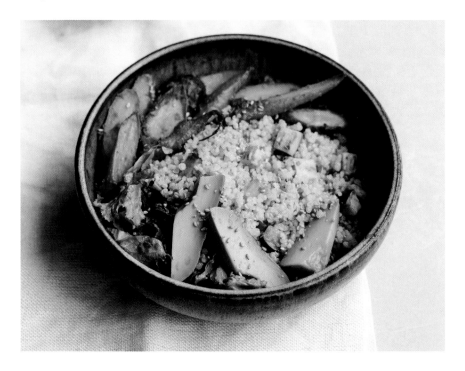

miso-glazed kabocha + carrots over brown rice bowl

Serves 2 in big bowls or 3 in small bowls

There is something magical about roasted squash and root veggies—it's that starchy, earthy sweetness, in this case mixed with savory tofu over hearty brown rice. This perfectly balanced recipe is made with a simple miso marinade, but feel free to swap in your favorite homemade dressing and top it off with some fresh greens.

MISO MARINADE

2 tablespoons toasted sesame oil

2 tablespoons organic red miso paste

2 tablespoons rice vinegar

½ teaspoon honey or pure maple syrup

GRAIN BOWL

3 cups leftover cooked brown rice (mix with sweet mochi rice, if possible, to keep the rice moist)

4 organic carrots, sliced on the bias into 1½-inch pieces (about 2 cups)

2 cups 1½-inch cubes unpeeled kabocha squash

TOPPINGS

2 cups fresh greens (your choice of arugula, chopped kale, mizuna, or red-leaf lettuce)

1 avocado, pitted, peeled, and sliced into 1-inch cubes

2 teaspoons gomashio or toasted sesame seeds

1 block organic extra-firm savory tofu, drained and patted dry, cut into ¾-inch cubes (about 2 cups; optional)

Preheat the oven to 375°F. Line a baking sheet with aluminum foil or parchment paper.

In a large bowl, add all the ingredients for the miso marinade and whisk well to combine.

Add the carrots and kabocha squash to the marinade and set aside for about 20 minutes.

Spread out the marinated carrots and kabocha on the prepared sheet in an even layer. Place on the middle rack of the oven and roast for 30 to 35 minutes. Remove from the oven and set aside to cool slightly.

Add the brown rice to your serving bowls and top off each bowl equally with the roasted veggies.

Finish the bowls with your choice of fresh greens, avocado cubes, and/or some toasted and ground sesame seeds or gomashio. Top with the tofu, if using.

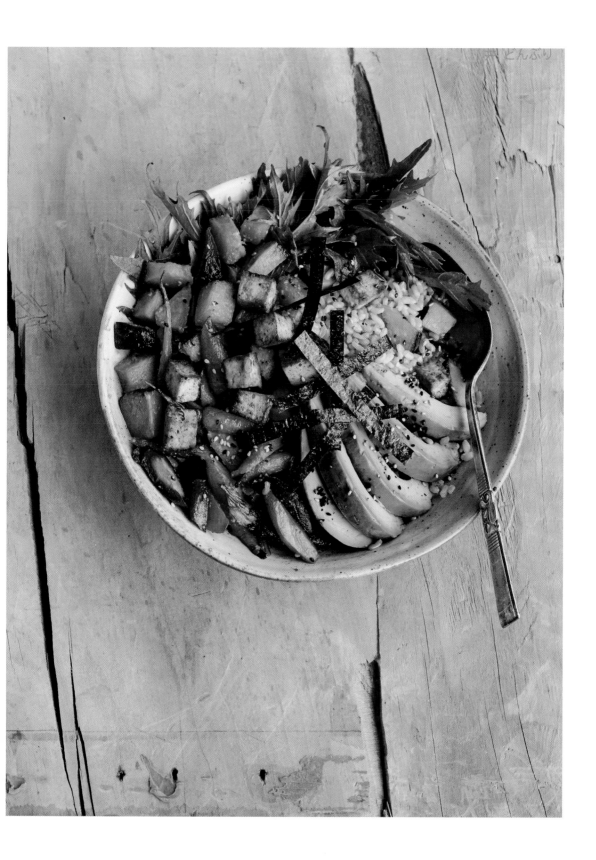

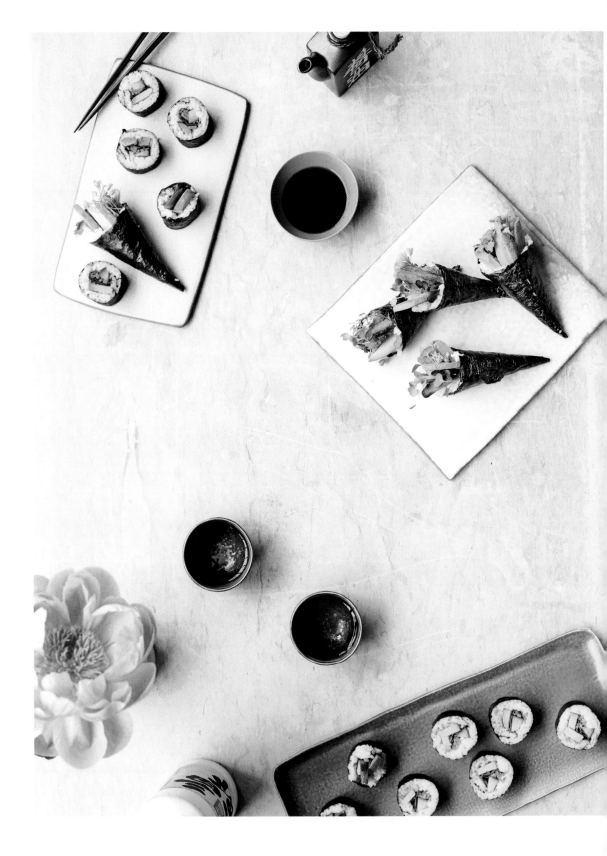

basics

基本，きほん

kihon

savory tofu

Serves 4

One of the things I love about tofu is that it takes on the flavor of whatever you cook it with. This basic tofu recipe produces a lightly seasoned, savory tofu you can add to almost any dish.

Nonstick olive or coconut oil cooking spray

¼ cup reduced-sodium tamari soy sauce

¼ cup rice vinegar

2 tablespoons mirin

2 to 3 garlic cloves, minced

One 14-ounce package organic firm tofu

In a medium storage container, combine the tamari soy sauce, rice vinegar, mirin, and minced garlic. Set aside.

Remove the block of tofu from its packaging and drain well, blotting the tofu with paper towels to remove excess liquid. Slice the tofu in half and then into 8 blocks, roughly 2 ounces per block. Place the blocks into your marinade, cover, and place in the fridge. Marinate the tofu for 15 minutes. Turn the tofu blocks and marinate for an additional 15 minutes.

Preheat the oven to 375°F. Line a baking sheet with aluminum foil and lightly coat with cooking spray.

Arrange the marinated tofu on the prepared sheet in an even layer. Bake for 20 minutes, remove from the oven, and set aside while preparing your meal.

kabocha no nitsuke shōyu aji (shōyu kabocha) 南瓜の煮付け醤油味, かぼちゃのにつけしょうゆあじ（醤油南瓜　しょうゆかぼちゃ）

Serves 4

In traditional Japanese culture okazu *refers to side dishes that are paired with rice.* Nitsuke *refers to simmered dishes.* Kabocha no Nitsuke *is my favorite okazu-style dish. The flavors marry beautifully, and while it is indeed traditional, it is also very simple to make!*

1 medium unpeeled kabocha squash

1 cup water

¼ cup plus 1 tablespoon reduced-sodium tamari soy sauce

¼ cup mirin

1 teaspoon organic sugar

Sriracha sauce, for seasoning (optional)

Leaving the skin intact, carefully cut your kabocha squash in half and remove all the seeds. Cut into quarters and then into 1-inch cubes. Set aside.

In a large stockpot (the bottom of the pan must be large), bring the water, tamari soy sauce, mirin, and sugar to a simmer over medium-low heat.

Add the kabocha cubes to the simmering liquid. Give it a stir and simmer for about 15 minutes, or until the kabocha is cooked through. Immediately remove the squash from the pot and transfer to a plate or bowl; do not leave the squash sitting in the liquid, or it will get mushy!

Serve as a side dish or over steamed brown rice with greens and a touch of sriracha sauce, if desired.

onigirazu
おにぎらず (sushi sandwiches)

Makes 6 sushi sandwiches

Need to pack a lunch or a snack that's not sweet, on the go? This "sushi" sandwich is the perfect and filling portable treat. It's one of my favorite ways to eat plant-based sushi out at the park, or when traveling. You can add everything from avocado to sweet potato, takuan pickles to spinach, all of your favorites, anything really goes. Don't forget to eat it on the same day, as the nori will soak into the rice after a few hours.

2 cups cooked rice (seasoned sushi rice or plain steamed rice)

6 nori sheets

2 sweet potatoes, cut into small wedges and roasted with 1 tablespoon coconut oil

1 avocado, pitted, peeled, and thinly sliced

1 cup thinly sliced purple cabbage (can also be pickled cabbage)

1 to 2 cups baby spinach, or your favorite greens

1 to 2 cups torn red-leaf lettuce

Sriracha sauce, as desired

Curry powder, just a sprinkle can add magic

Make the seasoned sushi rice (page 169). Or if you prefer plain, unseasoned rice, just add some sea salt to a bowl of water and use wet hands to shape the rice.

On top of a clean cutting board, place a nori sheet facedown and toward you in a diamond shape. Add about $1/3$ cup of the rice, pressing it firmly into the middle of your nori sheet.

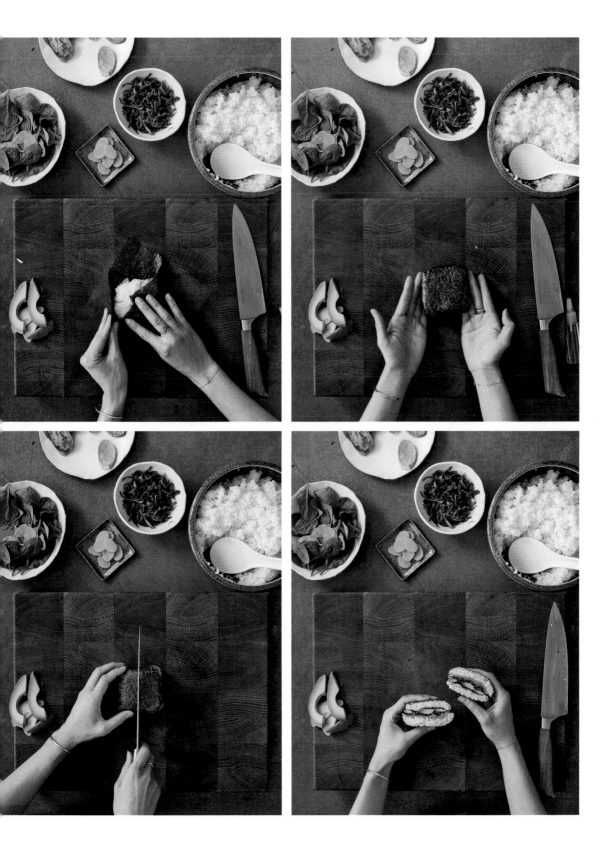

Add your choice of toppings in three or four layers, leaving a $^1/_2$-inch border of rice around the toppings.

With clean hands, add a final layer of sushi rice. Using a spray bottle, spritz some water onto the rice, then fold up the bottom tip of the nori, and fold all in sides as you would an envelope. If your nori is being naughty, spritz water onto it. Make sure your sandwich is tucked in tightly.

Flip the sandwich, place it in plastic wrap, and wrap it up like a sandwich (see images for reference). Keep your sandwich wrapped tightly in the plastic wrap and pack for a to-go lunch, or cut it into halves and eat immediately. So yum!

spicy avocado-cucumber maki rolls
巻き寿司, まきずし, makizushi

Serves 4; makes about 10 rolls or 60 pieces

Spicy avocado and crisp, fresh cucumbers make this my kind of California roll. The best part of making your own sushi at home is not only saving money, but having your rolls exactly how you like them. So feel free to personalize this recipe any way you want!

SUPPLIES

Bamboo mat

Rice paddle

Paper fan

Sharp knife

Clean, wet towel

SUSHI

10 to 12 sheets nori, toasted

2 cups uncooked sushi rice

SUSHI VINEGAR (SUSHI-SU) 寿司酢, すしす

¼ cup rice vinegar

3 tablespoons organic sugar

2 teaspoons sea salt

SPICY MAYO

3 tablespoons olive oil mayo or vegan mayo

3 tablespoons sriracha sauce

FILLING

2 ripe avocados, pitted, peeled, and thinly sliced lengthwise

2 medium cucumbers, sliced into thin strips

1 large or 2 medium carrots, sliced into thin julienne strips

2 cups baby spinach leaves

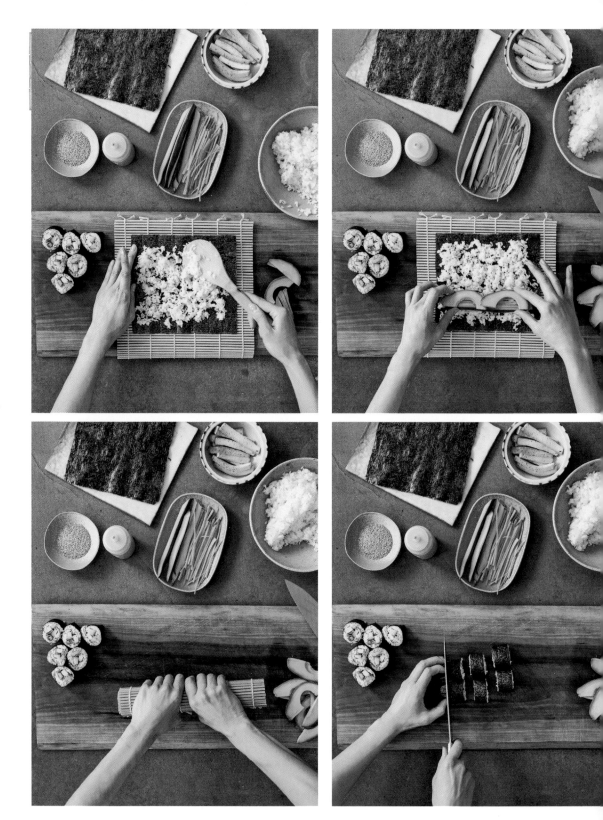

One to two 6-ounce packages organic firm savory tofu (like Wildwood brand; or make homemade savory tofu, see page 162), thinly sliced (optional)

OPTIONAL SEASONINGS

Reduced-sodium tamari soy sauce, for dipping

Ponzu sauce, for dipping

Sriracha sauce

Gomashio

Make the sushi rice: Wash your rice thoroughly and drain. Prepare and cook the sushi rice as directed on the package, or measure 2 cups sushi rice and cook with $2^1/_4$ cups water. Cool the rice slightly while preparing your sushi-su (sushi vinegar).

In a large bowl, combine the rice vinegar, sugar, and salt. Whisk well to dissolve the sugar and salt.

Transfer the slightly cooled sushi rice to the bowl with the sushi-su. Using a rice paddle and a cutting motion, distribute the sushi-su into the rice, coating the rice as you fan the rice to cool it at the same time. Be sure not to mix the rice. Simply cut through the rice until all the sushi-su is absorbed.

Make the spicy mayo: In a medium bowl, whisk the mayo and sriracha to incorporate; set aside.

Roll the sushi: While the rice is still warm, roll your sushi on a clean work surface, like a clean cutting board or a clean countertop. Lay your bamboo mat on the work surface. Place a nori sheet on top of the bamboo mat, shiny-side down.

Using your rice paddle, spread a layer of about $^1/_3$ cup of the seasoned sushi rice in the middle of the nori sheet, leaving a $^3/_4$-inch border all around. At the bottom of the sheet, closest to you, add your choice of fillers, placing them in a horizontal line toward the bottom of the roll:

2 avocado slices, 2 cucumber slices, 2 carrot slices, and a few baby spinach leaves. Drizzle the roll with 2 teaspoons of the spicy mayo.

Using the bamboo mat, tightly roll your sushi from the bottom up into a long roll. (Similar to how you would roll a baked jelly roll.) Gently squeeze the bamboo mat to tighten your roll. Unroll the mat.

Cut the roll as follows: Place your roll onto a clean cutting board. Using a sharp knife, cut your roll in half. (Wipe off your knife with a clean towel in between each slice.) Next, line up your two halves together and cut each into 3 equal pieces. Each roll should make 6 pieces.

Repeat until all the sushi rice is used.

Serve immediately, paired with a sake or Japanese beer.

maki = sushi roll
巻き寿司　まきずし
makizushi

Maki rolls are cut Japanese sushi rolls. Sushi was originally created as a way to preserve meat and fish before refrigeration. Eventually the Japanese started using vinegar to help the preservation process. And thus, over time, we have sushi:

nigiri sushi (fish over rice)
maki sushi (cut sushi rolls, wrapped in seaweed)
temaki sushi (hand rolls, wrapped in seaweed)

There are more kinds of sushi, like *inari-zushi*, *uramaki*, and *sashimi* (just the fish!), which I've embraced and loved since my childhood.

spicy avocado + curried carrot hand rolls temaki: 手巻き寿司 "temakizushi"

Makes about 18 hand rolls

I love adding a sprinkle of curry powder or turmeric to my temaki (hand rolls) for a little extra flavor. Once you've mastered the basics of making hand rolls, you can create as many varieties as you can imagine. The flavor combinations here are a good place to start!

HAND ROLLS

2 cups uncooked sushi rice or brown rice

10 to 12 nori sheets, toasted

SUSHI VINEGAR (SUSHI-SU) 寿司酢, すしす

¼ cup rice vinegar

3 tablespoons sugar

2 teaspoons organic sea salt

CURRIED CARROTS

4 medium carrots, thinly sliced on the bias

2 tablespoons unrefined coconut oil, melted

1 tablespoon curry powder

¼ teaspoon sea salt

SPICY AVOCADO HAND ROLL FILLERS

2 ripe avocados, pitted, peeled, and thinly sliced

2 cups baby spinach (optional)

One 2.5-ounce package kaiware (Japanese radish sprouts)

Sriracha sauce, as desired

Gomashio (optional)

Make the curried carrots: Preheat the oven to 375°F.

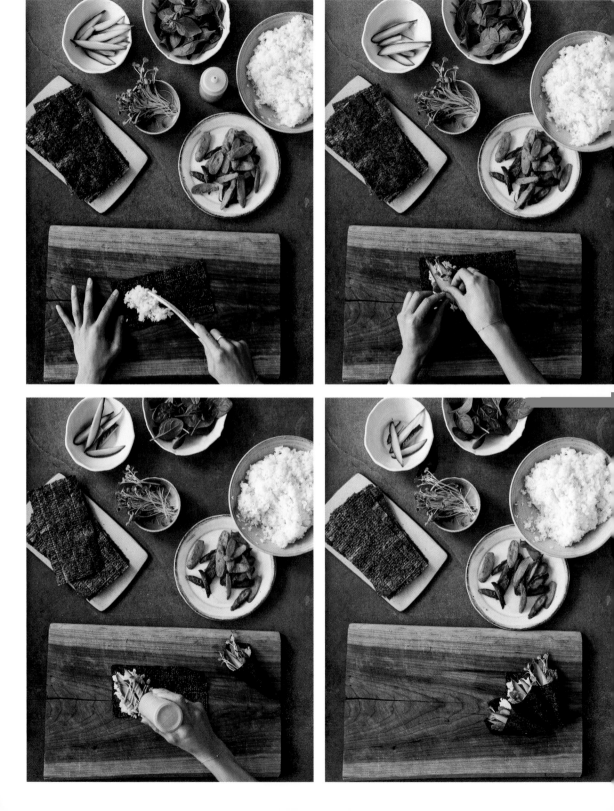

Place the carrots on a baking sheet, drizzle with the coconut oil, and sprinkle with the curry powder and sea salt. Toss to coat the carrots evenly. Roast the carrots for 30 minutes, then set aside to cool slightly.

Make the seasoned sushi rice: Wash the sushi rice thoroughly and drain. Prepare and cook the sushi rice as directed on the package, or measure 2 cups sushi rice and cook with $2^{1}/_{4}$ cups water. Cool the rice slightly while preparing your sushi vinegar.

In a large bowl, combine the ingredients for the sushi vinegar and whisk well to dissolve the sugar and salt.

Transfer the slightly cooled sushi rice into the same large bowl. Using a rice paddle and a cutting motion, distribute the sushi-su (vinegar) into the rice, coating the rice as you fan the rice to cool at the same time. Be sure not to mix the rice. Simply cut through the rice until all of the sushi-su is absorbed.

Fold the nori sheets in half and tear them to make 20 to 24 half sheets. Have a small bowl of room-temperature water ready.

On a clean surface, place a nori half in front of you (see image). Place about $^{1}/_{4}$ cup of the seasoned sushi rice diagonally on the bottom left corner of the nori sheet. Line up 2 to 4 curried carrot slices, avocado slices, kaiware sprouts (as seen in image), and fillers, if desired. Tightly roll the nori into a cone shape (see image) around the filling and seal the edge of the nori with a dab of water.

umeboshi potatoes

My super-creative and brilliantly talented cousin in Tokyo, Yukiko, showed me how to make the most simple ume mashed potatoes. They're now a staple on our Japanese American table for the holidays. **Domo arigatō** どうもありがとう**, Yukiko-san!**

5 large russet or Yukon Gold potatoes, peeled and cut into 2-inch cubes

2 to 4 umeboshi plums (depending on how you like it; 2 for subtle taste, 4 for slightly stronger), pitted

½ cup unsweetened almond milk

Sea salt (optional)

In a large stockpot or saucepan, boil the potatoes until slightly soft when tested with a fork. Carefully drain the potatoes, and return to the pot.

Using a potato masher, mash the potatoes with the umeboshi, looking for stray pits as you mash (be sure to remove them!). Add the almond milk and mix well to combine all the flavors. Season with a touch of salt, if desired.

Shizuko, age ninety-six; my grandmother's best friend has shared her home-made country umeboshi and her friend's various homemade recipes with us for decades. Umeboshi has a long shelf life, due to its preservation process, and is a total staple in the everyday Japanese life.

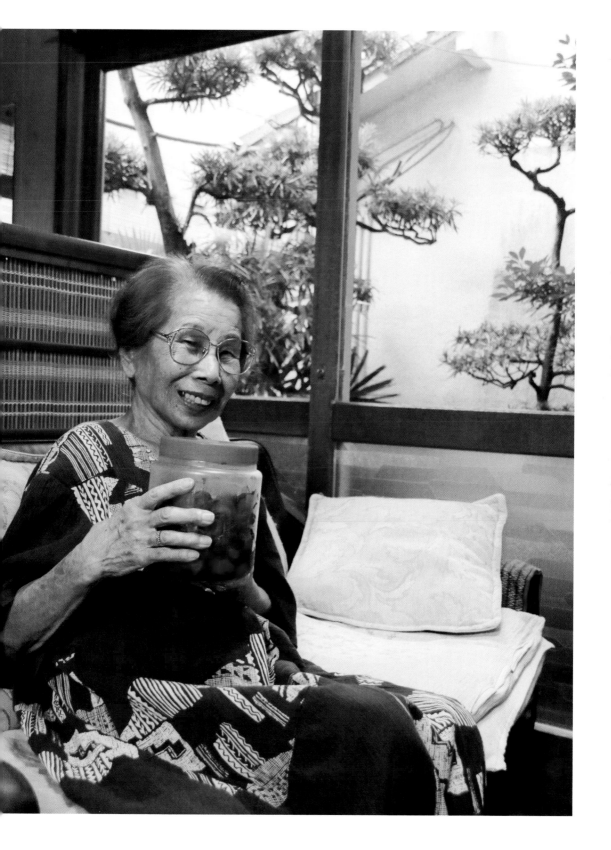

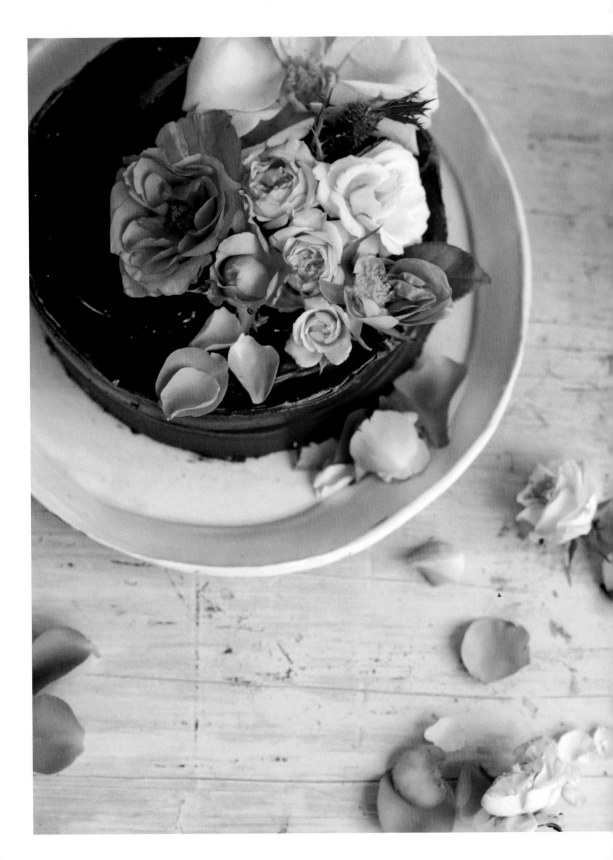

japanese-inspired sweets

和菓子, わがし

wagashi

matcha
抹茶, まっちゃ

I was introduced to matcha at a young age—around the same time my mom introduced me to sushi, ramen, udon, tsukemono, yakitori, and okonomiyaki. I can't even time-stamp it, because I was a little kid. But for me, matcha is an honorary treat and part of our Japanese heritage. Today, it's grown into a bona fide food trend and popular hashtag.

When I went to culinary school over a decade ago, I experimented with matcha and found ways to incorporate it into my crepes, pancakes, and baked goods. I began to appreciate the versatility of this traditional ingredient.

Years back, in Kyūshū, my Japanese mother gave Jenni and me my Baachan's matcha supplies, including her chasen (bamboo whisks). My Baachan and her youngest sister, my Auntie Takuko, studied tea and matcha under a tea master in Kyūshū. They were both around fifty years old when they seriously started to learn. (They have a saying in Japanese, *Gojū no tenarai*, "50 の 手習い、ごじゅう の てならい," meaning you start to learning something you really want after you are fifty years old.)

My Auntie Takuko took me to study matcha under a true tea master years ago, in her hometown of Beppu. I feel honored to be able to use my family's tools and traditions every time I whip up a cup of matcha. While matcha might be trending on social media, I am dedicated, along with many others, to keeping the integrity of this tradition intact. So here's a bit on one of my favorite Japanese ingredients:

In Japan traditional matcha at tea ceremonies was not mixed with sugar. The Japanese do enjoy sweets with matcha, like crepes, cakes, and even matcha chocolates. My mom shared with me that her first memory of matcha was *Ujikintoki* (*Uji matcha kakigori*; 宇治金時), shaved ice with sweet matcha syrup and sweet adzuki beans, sometimes with matcha ice cream! Yum!

The Westernization of matcha has turned it into a sweet treat, but traditionally matcha tea is made up of just two ingredients: ceremonial-grade matcha powder and water that is slightly under boiling.

To make matcha, boil water, and allow it to cool slightly, for just a few minutes (it should be between 175° and 185°F). Place sifted matcha powder into a clean and dry *chawan* matcha bowl. Add a small bit of the hot water to the bowl. Using a chasen (bamboo whisk), whisk up tiny, tiny bubbles, moving your whisk in vigorous M and N motions. When the matcha powder is fully incorporated and the tea is frothy, enjoy!

when purchasing matcha, here's what to look for:

Japanese-produced matcha powder is the way to go. I purchase my matcha direct from Japan (Uji, Shiga, Wazuka, Mie, Miyazaki are all great regions for the best matcha). In the States, Matcha Love by Ito En is a trusted source of Japanese teas. Always look for "ceremonial grade" and/or "product of Japan" on the label. Organic is always best.

When purchasing online, read reviews to make sure the brand is reputable. Also, keep in mind that plain matcha powder contains only powdered green tea—no sugar, no other ingredients.

Lastly, check the expiration date and make sure your matcha is fresh as possible before you purchase. Matcha will only last for about a year. You can store your matcha in a cool, dark place or in your refrigerator. Look for a bright green color when using.

matcha chocolate chip pancakes

Serves 4; makes 10 to 12 pancakes

When I really like someone, I offer to make them pancakes in the morning.
It's a staple in my household and a simple gesture to show someone I care.
Make these pancakes as a surprise for someone you love.

DRY INGREDIENTS

1½ cups gluten-free baking flour or all-purpose flour

2 tablespoons matcha powder

1½ teaspoons aluminum-free baking powder

WET INGREDIENTS

2 large eggs (optional)

2 tablespoons brown rice syrup, or organic sugar

1¼ to 1½ mashed ripe bananas

1 teaspoon organic vanilla extract

1 cup unsweetened almond milk

¾ cup high-quality dark chocolate chips

Coconut oil cooking spray

TOPPINGS

Kinako powder (see sidebar; optional)

Fresh fruit (optional)

Whisk the flour, matcha, and baking soda together in a large bowl. Set the dry ingredients aside.

In a separate medium bowl, whisk together the eggs (if using), brown rice syrup, banana, vanilla, and almond milk. Add the wet ingredients to the dry ingredients and gently whisk to combine. Using a rubber spatula, fold in the chocolate chips; the batter will be thick.

Lightly coat a large nonstick skillet with cooking spray and heat over medium heat. Using ¹/₄ cup of batter for each pancake and cooking two to three pancakes at a time, pour the batter into the skillet, cook the pancakes until the outer edges firm up and the bottoms are golden brown, about 2 minutes. Flip and cook the other side until golden brown, about 2 minutes more. Remove from the pan and set aside on a plate. Repeat with the remaining batter. Serve with a touch of kinako powder and fresh fruit, if desired!

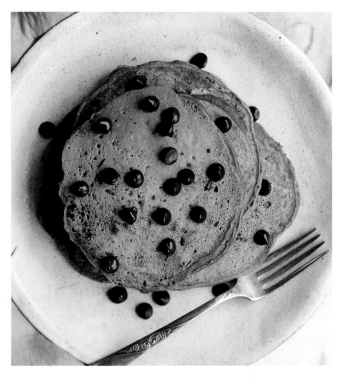

kinako powder: きな粉 きなこ

This wildly popular roasted soybean flour is a staple in Japanese households. Kinako is sprinkled over dango, mochi, ice cream, and pancakes, and you can even blend it into your smoothies. The earthy, rich flavor of kinako is what makes it so unique. Kinako is packed with plant protein, calcium, and iron. Every time I sprinkle this powdered goodness on my recipes, it takes me back to my childhood love of kinako over hot, fresh mochi! You can find kinako powder at your local Japanese grocery store. Mix about ½ cup kinako with 1 to 2 teaspoons organic sugar. Store in an airtight container in the fridge for up to 2 months.

matcha–chocolate chip cookies

Makes 18 to 20 cookies

These super-moist and delicious cookies were based on one of my most popular cookie recipes from my first book, Pretty Delicious. *They are made with a secret ingredient: banana! Pro tip: Try to resist eating them fresh out of the oven (I know, it's hard). They taste even better the next day!*

Nonstick olive or coconut oil cooking spray

¾ cup gluten-free flour

½ teaspoon aluminum-free baking powder

¼ teaspoon sea salt

3 tablespoons unrefined coconut oil, melted

1 teaspoon organic vanilla extract

⅓ cup organic sugar (or 5 drops of stevia)

1 egg (if making vegan, add 1 to 2 tablespoons of water)

1½ ripe medium bananas, mashed

½ cup organic rolled oats

1 cup semisweet chocolate chips

1 tablespoon matcha powder, sifted

Preheat the oven to 325°F. Line a rimmed baking sheet with aluminum foil and coat lightly with cooking spray.

In a medium bowl, whisk together the flour, baking powder, and salt; set aside.

In a large bowl, whisk together the coconut oil, vanilla, and sugar (or stevia) to combine. Add the egg (or water) and whisk well to incorporate.

Using a rubber spatula, scrape down the sides and bottom of the bowl as necessary. Mix in the mashed banana and stir until well incorporated.

Add the dry ingredients to the wet ingredients and stir until combined. Using a rubber spatula, fold in the oats and chocolate chips. Sprinkle in the sifted matcha powder and fold in gently.

Chill the cookie dough in the refrigerator for 15 minutes.

Using a tablespoon, scoop out $1^1/_2$-inch balls and place them about 1 inch apart on the prepared baking sheet. Bake until lightly golden on top, 10 to 13 minutes. Cool on the baking sheet for 5 minutes before transferring the cookies to a wire rack to cool completely.

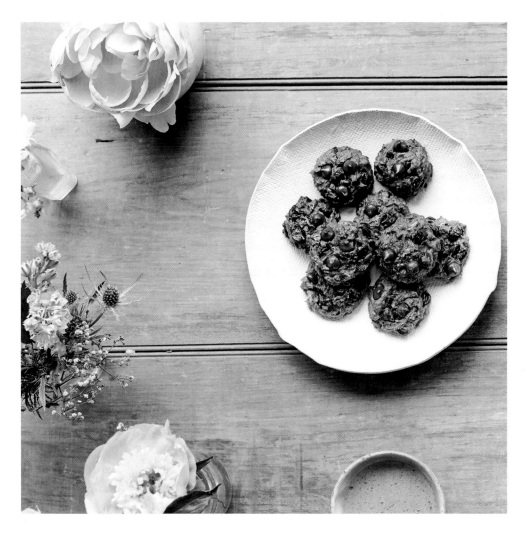

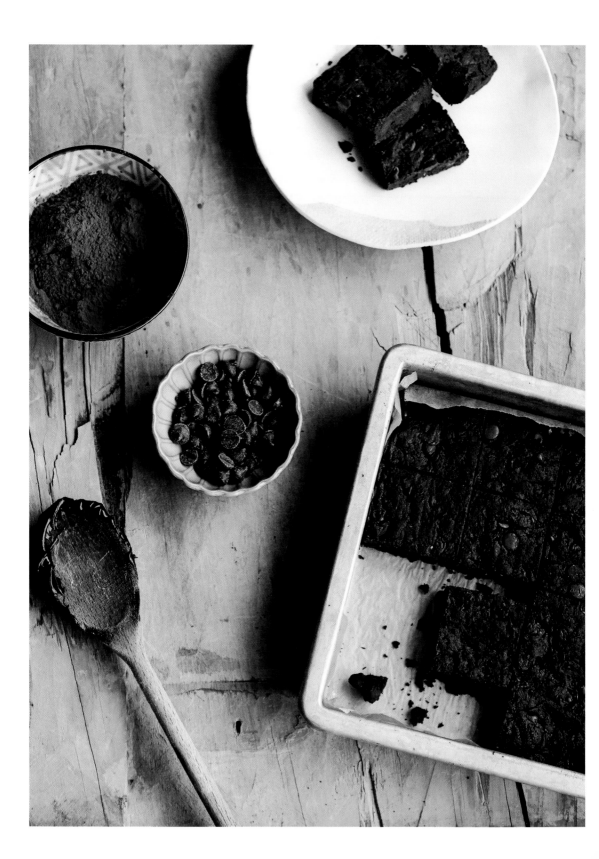

adzuki bean dark chocolate brownies

Makes 12 to 16 brownies

These dense, fudgy, decadent brownies are made with a secret ingredient:
adzuki beans!

WET INGREDIENTS

Nonstick olive or coconut oil cooking spray

1¼ cups cooked adzuki beans (if canned, rinsed and drained)

2 eggs plus 1 egg yolk

½ cup unrefined coconut oil, slightly melted

2 tablespoons water, as needed

⅓ cup packed organic sugar or coconut sugar

1 teaspoon organic vanilla extract

DRY INGREDIENTS

1 cup unsweetened dark cocoa powder

1 tablespoon cornstarch

1 teaspoon aluminum-free baking powder

¼ teaspoon sea salt

1½ cups dark chocolate chips

Preheat the oven to 325°F. Lightly coat an 8-inch square baking dish with cooking spray.

In a large bowl, mash the adzuki beans well with a fork. Add the eggs, oil, water, sugar, and vanilla. Whisk well to combine. Set the wet ingredients aside.

In a medium bowl, mix together the cocoa powder, cornstarch, baking powder, and salt. Slowly whisk the dry ingredients into the wet.

Using a rubber spatula, fold in chocolate chips until incorporated. Scrape the batter into the prepared baking dish and smooth the surface. Bake on the middle rack of the oven until the sides are set and pull away from the baking dish, 36 to 38 minutes. Remove from the oven and cool before serving.

matcha coconut ice cream

Serves 4

This dairy-free ice cream is one of my favorite treats, especially in the summer! Infused with matcha and a touch of organic vanilla, it has a rich, sweet flavor. I like to top mine with delish add-ons like chocolate chips, coconut, mint, or—best of all—sprinkles!! (As a child of the eighties, I still believe that sprinkles are best on everything.)

1 tablespoon high-quality matcha powder

Three 14-ounce cans full-fat coconut milk

¼ cup brown rice syrup or pure maple syrup

2 tablespoons high-quality vodka

1 teaspoon organic vanilla extract

TOPPINGS

Natural sprinkles (optional)

Dark chocolate chips (optional)

Fresh mint (optional)

Toasted coconut shavings (optional)

Place the matcha into a bone-dry, high-powered blender (like a Vitamix). Next, pour in the coconut milk, brown rice or maple syrup, vodka, and vanilla. Blend all the ingredients on high speed for at least a minute. The creamier the texture of the ice cream base, the better.

Pour the mixture into an ice cream maker and, following the machine's instructions, churn it up. When ready, serve immediately.

Store leftover ice cream in an airtight container in the freezer for up to 3 weeks. Note that this recipe is best when served fresh!

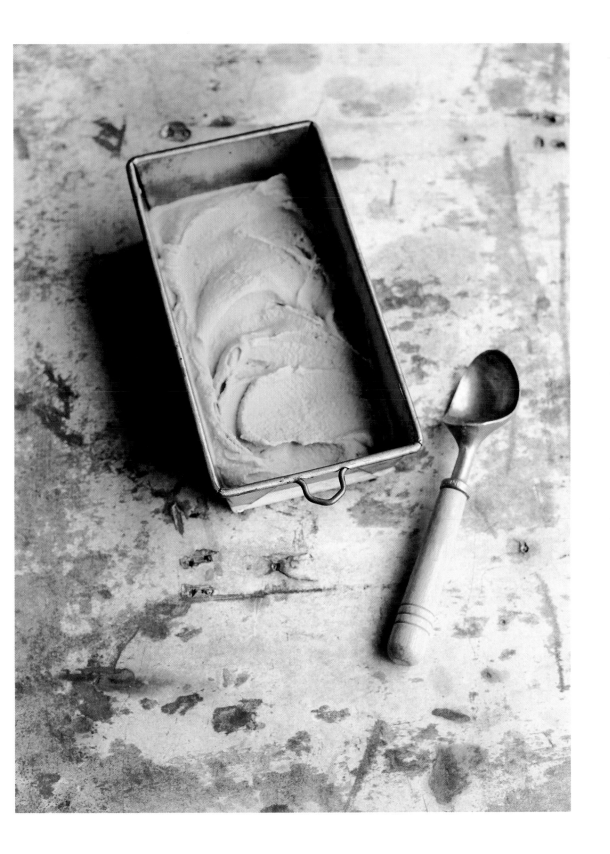

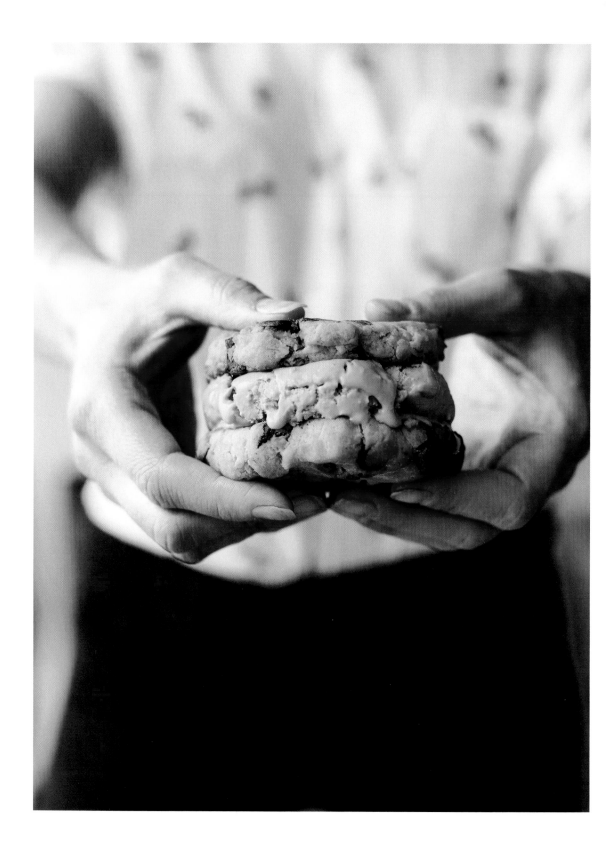

matcha ice cream sandwiches

Makes 4 ice cream sandwiches

These ice cream sandwiches are a nostalgic summer treat. I made these back in the Cali sun with friends, poolside—and every one of us felt like a kid again. I highly recommend making them for your next summer party!

8 large Matcha-Chocolate Chip Cookies (page 182) or Miso-Chocolate Chip Cookies (page 198)

2 to 4 cups Matcha Coconut Ice Cream (page 186)

½ cup natural sprinkles

Line up 4 of the cookies on a clean work surface. Using a large spoon or an ice cream scooper, add the ice cream to fill each "sandwich." Add another cookie on top.

Place the rainbow sprinkles on a shallow plate, and roll the exposed ice cream on the edges of the sandwich in the sprinkles. Or sprinkle them directly on the sandwiched ice cream, if desired.

Immediately and carefully wrap the sandwiches in plastic wrap and place in the freezer for 20 to 30 minutes to solidify. Enjoy immediately!

matcha dark chocolate–dipped scones

Makes 8 to 12 scones

These deliciously delicate matcha scones are perfection dipped in rich, dark chocolate. Feel free to sprinkle some slivered almonds or toasted coconut on the chocolate before it dries for extra-pretty scones.

SCONES

Coconut oil cooking spray

2 cups gluten-free flour, plus extra for rolling out dough

1 teaspoon aluminum-free baking soda

2 tablespoons matcha powder

¼ teaspoon sea salt

½ cup unrefined coconut oil, melted

1 large egg

½ cup unsweetened applesauce

¼ cup brown rice syrup

1 large egg yolk, beaten, for egg wash

2 tablespoons turbinado sugar (optional)

TO FINISH

¾ cup dark chocolate chips

slivered almonds or toasted coconut (optional)

Preheat the oven to 350°F. Line a baking sheet with aluminum foil and spray with cooking spray.

In a large bowl, combine the flour, baking soda, matcha powder, and sea salt.

In a separate large bowl, whisk together the coconut oil, egg, applesauce, and brown rice syrup. Add the dry ingredients to the wet ingredients and mix until a dough forms.

Turn the dough out onto a floured work surface and lightly flour your hands. Gently knead the dough, just until all the flour is incorporated. Mold the dough into a 1-inch-thick disk. Cut into 8 to 12 wedges (like a pie).

Transfer the scones to the prepared baking sheet. Brush with egg wash and sprinkle with the turbinado sugar, if desired. Bake on the middle rack until golden brown and baked through, about 14 minutes; cool completely.

Melt dark chocolate chips over a double boiler. Dip scones in melted dark chocolate or drizzle with the chocolate; allow the chocolate to set, sprinkle with toppings if desired.

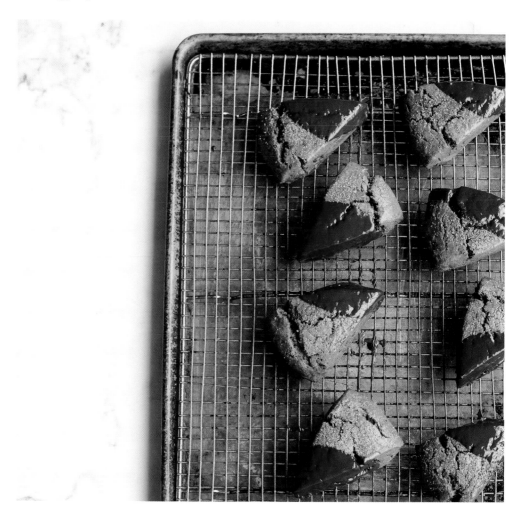

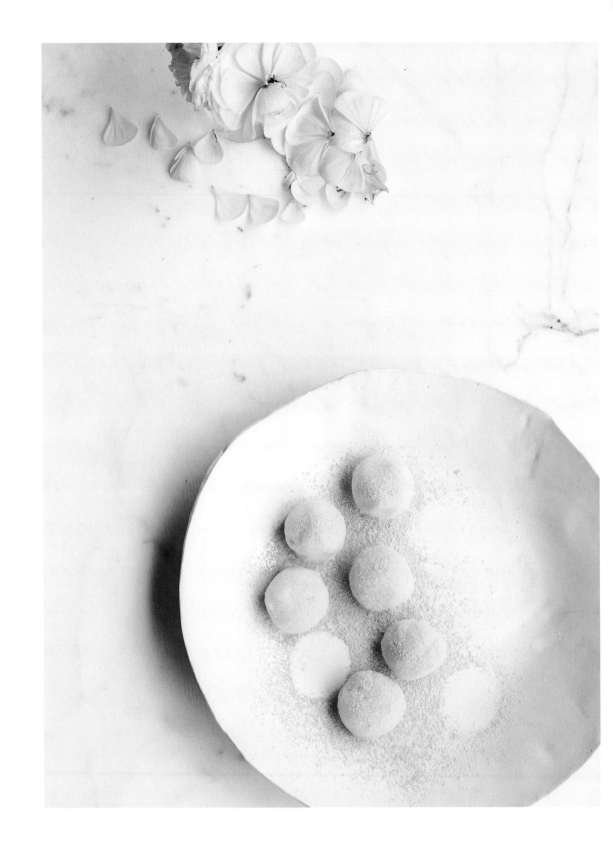

easy kinako dango
きな粉団子, きなこだんご

Makes about fifteen 1½-inch balls

This super-chewy and delish recipe is as close to real Japanese mochi as you can get! With the use of rice flour and a touch of silken tofu to make the dango soft, you'll love this satisfying treat! Top them off with kinako powder, and serve fresh off the stovetop.

½ cup organic silken tofu

½ cup plus 2 tablespoons boiling water

1½ cups Mochiko brand rice flour

½ cup kinako

1½ tablespoons organic sugar

Make the dough: In a large bowl, whisk the silken tofu well until well mashed. Carefully add the hot water and rice flour into the bowl and whisk well to incorporate. Let cool.

After mixture has cooled, with clean hands, form the mixture into a soft dough. Roll the dough into small $1^1/_2$-inch balls.

Bring a medium pot of water to a boil. Carefully add the dough balls to the boiling water and cook until they float to the top. Once the dango balls rise to the top, allow them to cook for an additional 1 to 2 minutes. Remove with a slotted spoon, shaking off any excess water. Place into serving bowls. In a small bowl, mix the kinako and sugar. Sprinkle the dango with the kinako-sugar mixture as pictured, and enjoy by eating immediately with your hands or with a fork!

sweet potato–turmeric loaf cake

Makes one 8-inch loaf cake

This delicious, fresh loaf bread is a perfect weekend treat with a touch of real butter or apple butter slathered on top. I created this lightly sweet bread with the intent of getting more turmeric into our diets and for you to enjoy more ukon—like the Okinawans do!

Coconut oil or olive oil cooking spray

3 large eggs, beaten

¼ cup organic sugar

⅓ cup unrefined coconut oil, melted

3 tablespoons light coconut milk

1 teaspoon organic vanilla extract

½ cup canned 100% pure sweet potato puree

1¼ cups rice flour

¾ teaspoon ground cinnamon

¾ teaspoon ground turmeric

1 teaspoon aluminum-free baking powder

¼ teaspoon sea salt

Preheat the oven to 350°F. Spray a small 8 x 4-inch loaf pan with cooking spray.

In a large bowl, whisk together the eggs and sugar. Whisk in the coconut oil, coconut milk, vanilla, and sweet potato puree. Slowly whisk in the rice flour, cinnamon, turmeric, baking powder, and sea salt.

When fully combined, pour the batter into the prepared loaf pan and bake for about 35 minutes, or until the center of the cake springs back to the touch. Cool and slice. Store in an airtight container for up to 1 week.

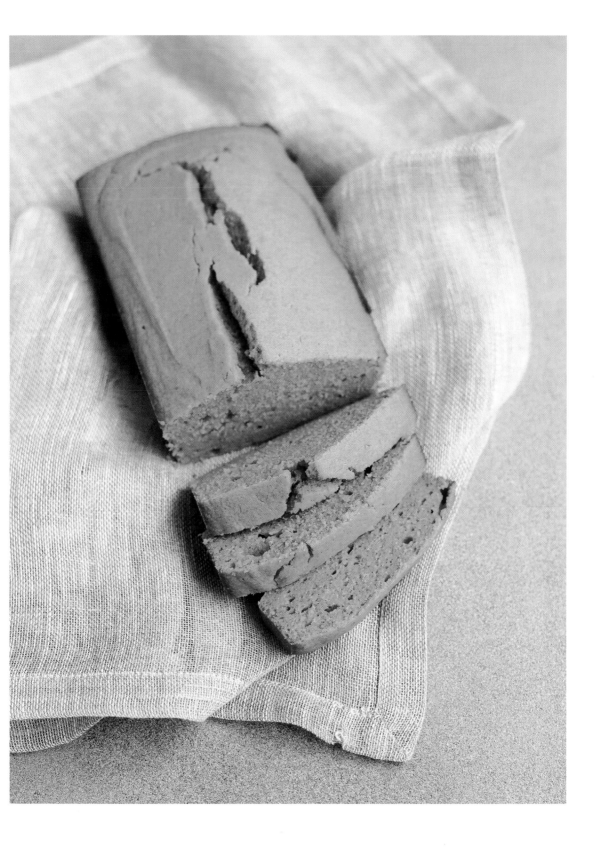

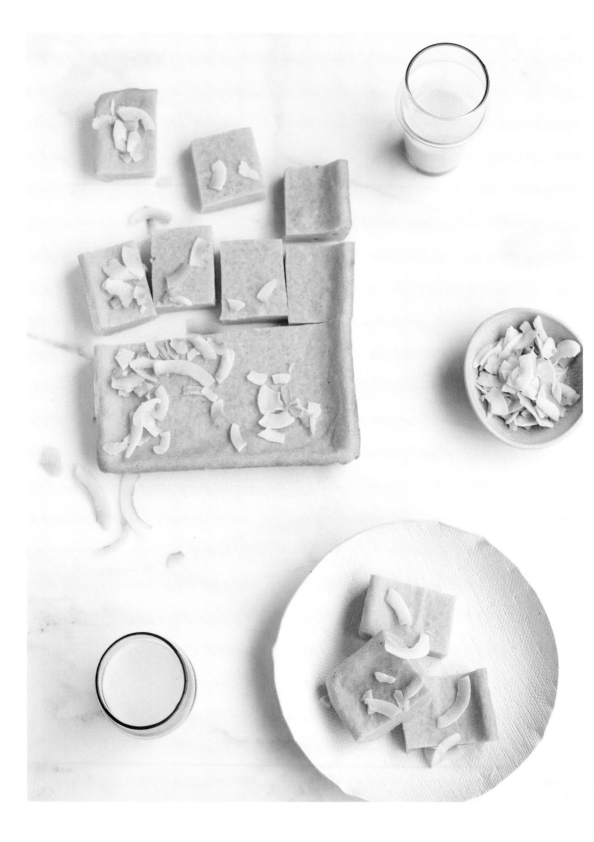

coconut mochi squares

Serves 18

When I was a kid, we used to go to the local Japanese Obon and Hanamatsuri festivals every year, and I always sought out this insanely delish mochi treat with a sesame seed crust. It was to die for. I still proudly have my sweet tooth, but I've made an effort to lower the sugar in this recipe (and many other desserts) so the indulgence is a little bit healthier.

Coconut oil or olive oil cooking spray

⅓ cup organic sugar

4 large eggs

½ cup unrefined coconut oil, melted

1 teaspoon organic vanilla extract

One 13.5-ounce can coconut milk

3 cups Mochiko brand mochi rice flour (sweet rice flour)

1 teaspoon aluminum-free baking powder

TOPPINGS

½ cup kinako, mixed with a touch of organic sugar

Toasted unsweetened coconut (optional)

Preheat the oven to 350°F. Coat a 9 x 13-inch baking dish with cooking spray.

In a medium bowl, whisk together the sugar, eggs, coconut oil, vanilla, and coconut milk until combined. Add the mochi flour and baking powder and fold in well using a rubber spatula. Scrape the batter into the prepared baking dish.

Bake for 33 to 35 minutes, until lightly golden at the top and cool in the pan.

After bars have slightly cooled, add a dusting of kinako or toasted coconut flakes to top.

miso–chocolate chip cookies

Makes 16 to 20 cookies

These soft cookies are my take on a salted chocolate treat. As I tested them with my friends, everyone kept asking, "What is in these cookies!?" To everyone's surprise, it's the touch of salty-sweet miso paste makes these cookies so addictive!

Nonstick olive or coconut oil cooking spray

⅓ cup organic sugar

½ cup unrefined coconut oil, melted

1 teaspoon organic vanilla extract

½ cup organic red or white miso paste (reduced-sodium miso is best)

2 large eggs

1 ½ cups gluten-free flour

½ teaspoon baking soda

1 cup dark chocolate chips

Preheat the oven to 325°F. Line a baking sheet with aluminum foil and coat with cooking spray.

In a medium bowl, whisk the sugar and coconut oil well to combine. Add the vanilla and miso paste and whisk well. Add the eggs and whisk gently to combine.

Using a rubber spatula, fold in the flour and baking soda and mix to combine the wet and dry ingredients. Fold in the chocolate chips.

Using a small ice cream scoop, scoop the cookies onto the prepared baking sheet, spacing them slightly apart.

Bake the cookies for 12 to 13 minutes. Remove from the oven and transfer to a wire rack to cool slightly. Store the cookies in an airtight container for up to 1 week.

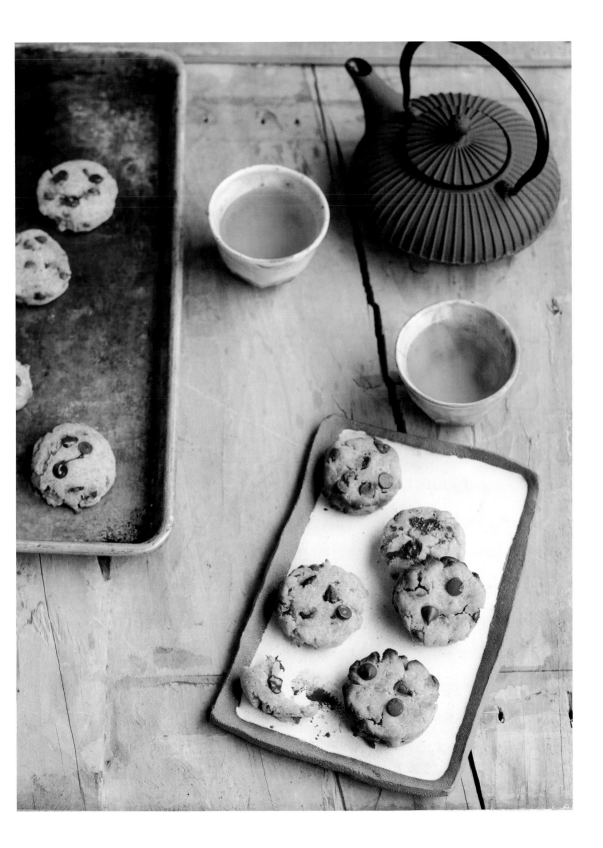

matcha dark chocolate cake

Makes one 8- or 9-inch cake; serves 12

This gorgeous vegan cake was much harder to perfect than I had originally anticipated. I worked on it for months, but I think I've finally gotten it pretty close to perfect. I've made it for birthdays, weddings, and dinner parties, and everyone asks for seconds! Remember, as Julia Child once said, "A party without a cake is just a meeting."

CAKE (Double recipe for 2-layer cake)

Coconut oil cooking spray

1 ripe banana, mashed well

¾ cup organic sugar

¾ cup unrefined coconut oil

1 teaspoon organic vanilla extract

1 cup water

2½ cups gluten-free flour (such as Bob's Red Mill for the best results)

1 cup almond flour

2 tablespoons cornstarch

¼ teaspoon sea salt

1 tablespoon matcha powder, sifted

1 teaspoon baking soda

1 tablespoon apple cider vinegar

DARK CHOCOLATE COCONUT FROSTING FOR TWO-LAYER CAKE (Frosting yields enough for two cakes)

2¾ cups confectioners' sugar, sifted

1½ cups dark unsweetened cocoa powder, sifted

½ cup plus 2 to 3 tablespoons coconut milk (canned or drinkable works), depending on how thick or smooth you like it

Make the cake: Preheat the oven to 350°F. Lightly coat an 8- or 9-inch round cake pan with cooking spray. Cut a round of parchment paper to fit the bottom of the pan, if desired (this helps to prevent the cake from sticking).

In a medium bowl, combine the mashed banana, sugar, and coconut oil, mix in the vanilla and water, and whisk well to combine.

In a small bowl, gently whisk together the gluten-free flour, almond meal–flour, cornstarch, and sea salt. Add the sifted matcha powder last. Mix using a whisk until combined, but do not overmix. Add the baking soda and apple cider vinegar, and fold in well.

Immediately pour the batter into the prepared cake pan and place on the lower rack of the oven. Bake for approximately 26 minutes.

Remove from the oven and cool completely prior to frosting the cake.

Make the frosting: In a large bowl, whisk together the confectioners' sugar, unsweetened cocoa powder, and coconut milk until fluffy and creamy.

Frost the cooled cake with half the frosting and store the rest in an airtight container in the fridge for up to three days.

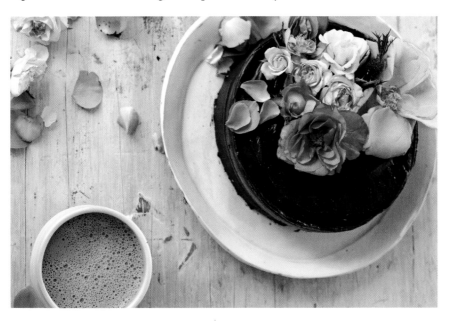

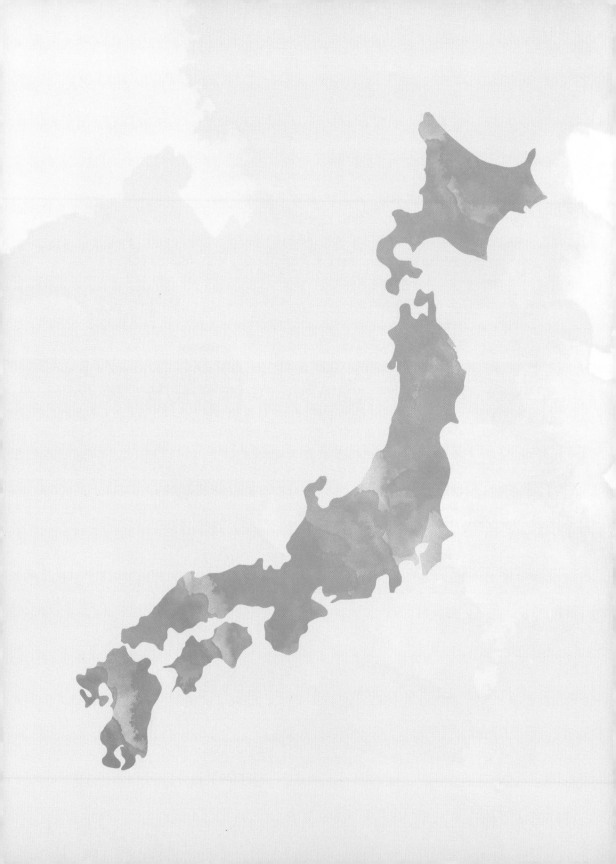

lifestyle
kurashikata

ライフスタイル

暮らし方, くらしかた

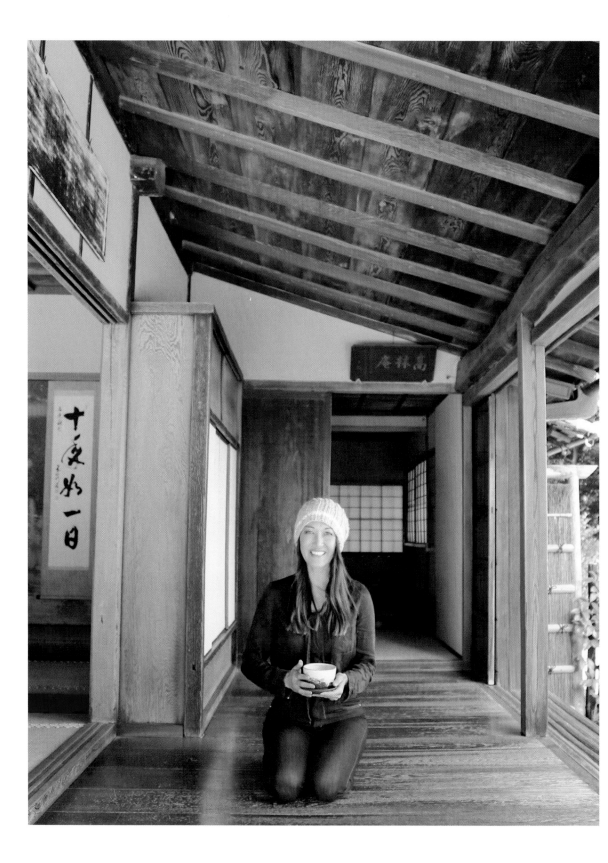

5

ki o tsukete

気をつけて

take care

WHENEVER I LEFT THE HOUSE AS A KID, MY MOM WOULD ALWAYS SAY, "*KI O TSUKETE NE!*," which let me know she cared about me in her strong and powerful way. A very common saying in Japan, ki o tsukete has many meanings: "Take care," "Be kind to yourself," "Pay attention."

In Japanese culture, whenever we speak about caring for others, we always use this phrase. It's very common for mothers to say it to their children, as my mom did. But we also say it to each other when we are parting ways, especially when sending family, friends, or colleagues off on a new endeavor. You are both wishing them well and encouraging them to be mindful of their surroundings.

When my mom used this phrase, she was really saying, "Pay attention! Stand tall. Head up, focus, drive, be strong." She could be hard on my sister and me, but these words of tough love and encouragement were actually her way of communicating to us that we were capable and therefore needed to show up.

Ki o tsukete is not an empty phrase used lightly; it is only said with sincerity. One of the things that struck me most about my time in Japan was the sincerity of daily communications. Whether you are engaging with a loved one or a stranger, the Japanese people make you feel like you're the most important person in the world. It felt quite different than the interactions I'm used to in my New York life.

How you interact with the world has a lot to do with how you make people feel. Sincerity makes people feel good, and it isn't something you can fake. Learning to be sincere is a lifelong practice, and one worth working on.

The only way I've found to cultivate sincerity is to spend more quiet time alone, looking inward. Becoming aware of how others feel starts with becoming more aware of how you feel. My mom taught me the importance of taking great care of myself and others. That is the heart of ki o tsukete.

take good care of you

Remember the airplane rule: Put on your own oxygen mask before helping others. It may sound selfish, but hear me out. Before we can nourish others, we must first take care of ourselves. For so long, I prioritized the needs of other people (friends, boyfriends, colleagues) without investing in the same care for myself. Some days, does it feel like everyone needs something from you? It can be exhausting, being connected to people 24/7. There are days when I wish e-mail did not exist.

It makes me feel good to take care of the people I love, but when you're not putting that same energy back into yourself, it can become draining.

Ki o tsukete reminds me to also take good care of myself, to pay attention, stand tall, be independent—all the things Mom always told me. For so many years working as a writer, I was focused on achievement and perfection. It took me a very long time to realize that I was nurturing the wrong goals. I needed to take care of my spirit and my physical body. When I finally began to shift my sails, things did indeed change for the better. My recipes became my very best, my heart felt full of gratitude, my writing became more personal. I was able to connect on a deeper level. But in order to get there, I had to practice more self-awareness, had to pay a great deal of attention, had to apply the essence of ki o tsukete to my life.

One way to understand the philosophy of ki o tsukete is to practice gratitude. Even on my toughest days, I'll remind myself to find three to five things to be grateful for, and often this list will snowball into ten to twenty. Sometimes I start with the simple fact that I have a strong body, a beating heart, and an active mind. I can create anything. I'm grateful for the people in my life, for the opportunities that have come my way. Whenever I focus on gratitude, my problems always feel more manageable. I encourage you to try this practice, as it will help you appreciate your good fortune and alleviate your worries.

don't be afraid to edit

I've spent a tremendous amount of my time caring for many different friends. I used to think it was customary to offer up equal amounts of friendship. But over the years, I began to realize that not everyone cared for me in the same way, not everyone reciprocated the same investment of energy and compassion.

By taking the time to care for myself, I became better able to judge which relationships felt essential to my well being, and which ones I could safely let go. When I understood my own needs with sincerity, I became more aware of how each interaction made me feel. Self-awareness led to self-respect, and I set clear boundaries around my space and my heart. If you give less energy to things that aren't worth it, you'll be able to open your heart to new things, new people, new friends, and new relationships. It's simple math: You are able to add more to your life when you've subtracted something.

It may seem like we need to stay in touch with everyone, forever, but relationships evolve. As our lives change, so do the people in them. The measure of any friendship is simple: How does it make you feel? If the answer is "not great," clean house. Don't be afraid to un-follow, let go, and take better care of you. When you edit who takes up space in your life, you'll begin to attract the right kind of people into your circle—those who are sincerely invested in your health and happiness.

trust yourself

Another part of ki o tsukete is the idea of being independent and trusting your own decisions. When I was first starting out in my career, so many people told me what to write, how to act, what to wear, what to cook, who to hang with, what to say. Naturally, I was tempted to go down a path laid out for me by someone else. Yet, deep inside, I knew I had to forge my own way.

A wise therapist once told me, "Don't let your true persona move far from who you are as a person," meaning, make sure your actions and what you do on the outside is in alignment with what you really believe. Your gut, your intuition will always guide you in the right direction. Trust yourself.

I'm proud to have been raised with tough love by immigrant parents. They gave my sister, Jenni, and me the gifts of freedom, independence, and wisdom. They made me who I am. During the coldest months in New York City, I'll often put my hand on my heart when I need Mom and Dad with me. I connect to the rhythm of my heart's beat (Mom and Dad), and say the words to myself: *Ki o tsukete*. Let these words comfort you, give you strength, and ground you, wherever you may be.

focus on the good stuff

Self-care has been a lifelong process for me, and it has not been easy. Like many women, I have struggled on and off with depression since adolescence. At some point, we all struggle with life's ups and downs. It can be hard to understand what is going on in your mind and body when you feel the lows particularly hard. But depression is also a part of who we are; it's only human.

When I am able to pause and reflect on the gifts in my life, doing so stops me from getting caught in a cycle of negative thoughts. This is the spiritual side of practicing ki o tsukete. Be mindful of how you talk to yourself, of the thoughts that are running through your mind. As much as possible, try to talk to yourself as you would a best friend—with positivity, love, and understanding. Honor yourself.

Counting your blessings—appreciating the ways in which you are self-sufficient instead of ruminating or pouting or feeling sorry for yourself—helps create the space to do good for others. I've found being of service to others helps me to feel more positive. Whether it's volunteering, doing a favor for a friend, or baking a cake or cookies to brighten someone's day, helping others always boosts my mood. Right now, more than ever, the world needs more people to step up and be of service to others.

lessons from okinawa

If there is one place in Japan where ki o tsukete is thriving, it's Okinawa. The southernmost island of Japan, is sometimes referred to Okinawa as the "Hawaii" of Japan. Prior to becoming part of Japan, Okinawa was its own nation. The island was occupied by Japan in 1879, by the United States in 1945, and finally reverted back to Japan in 1972.

Okinawans share a deep love and respect for nature—for the sunshine, local produce, the bounty of the sea. They are known for their healthy diet, low-stress lifestyle, and for their longevity. Okinawa is considered a "blue zone," which my friend Dan Buettner has researched for years. Dan's Okinawan and Japanese research on these "blue zones" has been inspiring to millions of us who read his books. Five times as many Okinawans live past the age of one hundred than people in the rest of Japan—and Japan is already ranked as one of the longest-living nations. Here is some of the wisdom I learned firsthand from my time there.

learn to adapt (tekiō; 適応 てきおう)

The Okinawans are experts at adaptation. During my time in Okinawa, I was given a tour of the caves where the Okinawans hid during World

War II. They showed me various war sites and shared personal stories of having nothing to eat but *satsuma-imo* (sweet potato). They told me survival stories about frantic escapes to the mainland.

My friend Mari, whom I met in Okinawa, was kind enough to introduce me and my sister to her grandparents, eighty-nine-year-old Nobu and eighty-eight-year-old Yoshiko Inafuku, who both shared with us the story of the final and deadly battle of the war in Okinawa. Nobu was only sixteen years old. He told me about the day where everything started out fine—the birds were chirping, the clouds were in the blue sky, and all was well. Then the U.S. ships came, and everything changed. He worked hard, as the oldest child, to keep the family together.

At the same time, his later-to-be wife, Yoshiko, was a young girl, only fifteen at the time. She shared with me that she and her family had to escape on a boat to Kyūshū, mainland Japan, to survive. Can you imagine how brave she was? The boat that left before hers, carrying over one thousand people, was bombed, and she was terrified. She got on the next boat and made it to the mainland. They told me how important it was, after living through the horrors of war, to have a positive outlook and a strong mind.

My conversations with Yoshiko and Nobu helped me to better understand what struggle was like at that time. Our problems seem so much smaller when we learn about what others, including our own ancestors, have gone through.

I then asked my friend Yoshiko how we can practice the strength and character of Okinawans. Her answer? "It's better to be happy all the time." One thing that touched me the most during my time in Okinawa was the repetition of this idea. I heard such deep stories, about war, tragedy, and

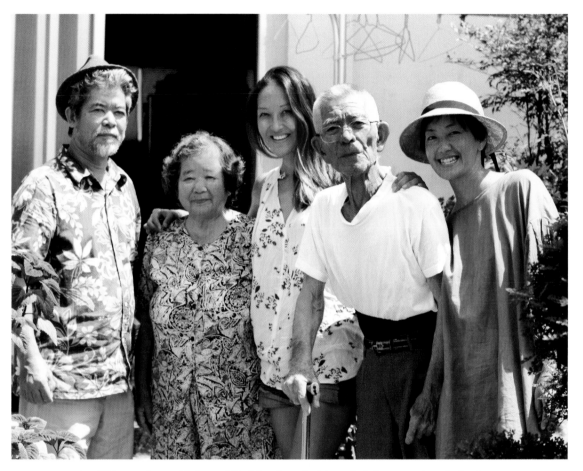

Okinawa, Japan: Nobu and Yoshiko shared with us their brave stories of what it was like living through World War II in Okinawa.

outcome that weren't fair. But no matter what these elders shared with me, they said they chose to be happy. Our mind-set is a choice, they explained. Instead of ruminating on what hasn't gone well for them, they instead choose to be happy.

A few months after I interviewed the Inafuku family, Mari and I

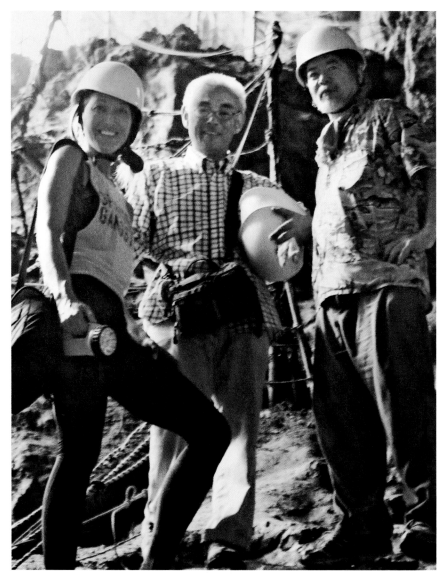

Okinawa, Japan: My guide Isao Oike-san is an incredible Japanese historian, and he, along with Uncle Tetsu (son of Nobu and Yoshiko Inafuku), showed my sister and me many caves across Okinawa in which thousands of Okinawans had to take refuge during the war.

reconnected, and she expressed her gratitude for the interviews with her grandparents. She was sad to share that her grandpa, Nobu Inafuku, had suddenly passed away. But because of our conversations, she had been able to learn more about her family history. I am so grateful to have met Nobu and Yoshiko, and will always honor their stories.

learn to be one with nature (shizen; 自然 しぜん)

Nature is available to everyone. No matter what part of the world you're in, nature is accessible and free. Spending time in the natural world heals us. Many of us are stuck inside at our jobs all day, but we can find small ways to incorporate more time spent outdoors. Take the long walk home from the bus or train stop, plan a weekend hike with friends, plan a trip to go camping at the beach, or visit a national park on your next vacation.

If you're short on space or access to the outdoors, incorporating more nature can be as easy as planting an herb garden outside your window! Space is tight for me in New York City, but I've managed to schedule in bike rides, runs, and long walks along the water. I've also packed my place with plants and fresh flowers from the local market. Whenever I can, I'll try to meet a friend in the park and gaze up at the trees all day. Sometimes, I'll save up for a trip to San Francisco or back home to San Diego. Spending time in nature is part of my self-care routine, and it feels really good.

Whether it means a simple meditation, sitting in a patch of sunshine in your apartment, or picking up some fresh-cut flowers at the farmers' market, find a moment to engage with the natural world each day. You can even visit nearby community garden to help others while simultaneously helping yourself!

The Okinawans prize the soil on which they live. Similarly, we should honor the gifts our earth has given us.

learn to cook! (ryōri! 料理. りょうり)

What's one main reason why so many Okinawans live so long? They grow, cook, and eat real food. The vast majority of Okinawans still make every meal from scratch, each and every day.

From a practical standpoint, Okinawans have traditionally grown all their own food because importing food to an island isn't easy. World War II also created a serious food shortage, and meat became unavailable. The resulting plant-based diet may be what has solidified the Okinawans' place among the world's longest-living people.

My friend Yoshiko, at age eighty-eight, tells me her secret to aging well is *imo*, otherwise known as the sweet potato! (Some of my favorite recipes for the magical sweet potato can be found on pages 98 and 142.) When you grow and cook your own food, you are taking a major step in caring for yourself. You will be able to see and feel the difference. And when you feel good, your whole life starts to improve.

every day is a good day (hibi kore kōjitsu)

I asked my friend Hiromi, who has lived in Okinawa for over twenty-five years, "What is it that keeps the women of Okinawa so vibrant and alive?" She didn't have to hesitate with her answer: "They work!"

Okinawan women have a lot to do. From the time they are very young, they get married, begin to take care of the farm, the family, and the community. But no matter how much there is to do, or how much they have to think about, they never seem to get overwhelmed. They focus on the positive, keep their eyes on the task at hand, and get things done. (Sound familiar?)

There's a Japanese phrase for this: *kodawaranai*, which translates to "Don't get so caught up in it." The simple meaning? Don't sweat the small stuff. Practice peace. Take care of what matters.

I've been a writer for over ten years, and most of the hours of my day are spent working. As a small business owner, I love working for myself in PJs, but I am responsible for paying my bills and paying my team. It's a balance. There's loads of administrative stuff to take care of, and sometimes I'd rather gag than do it. But it's my responsibility as a boss. There are also a lot of financial struggles that come along with the terrain. But when our work is meaningful to us, and when we bring our best selves to our jobs, every day is a good day.

be active! (アクティブ)

Okinawans are dedicated to movement well into their eighties and nineties. Each day I spent in Okinawa, I would get up at 5:00 or 6:00 a.m. to run, and would be amazed to see the local Okinawans out farming in the early mornings, in eighty-five degree heat! They were moving their bodies, farming their crops, making pottery, singing, dancing, all of it! In the afternoons, I watched them walk to the farmers' market to shop for fresh food. I even saw them walking to a community festival late into the night! It is their belief that you must physically move your body every twenty minutes or so to push aging away.

Unlike in the West, where we often equate physical activity with going to the gym, we can all learn from the ways Okinawans incorporate movement into their daily routines. One of my favorite things is how many elders ride their bikes around town. It's very common and always makes me smile. Try to incorporate this practice into your life in organic ways, whether it's walking more each day, parking your car farther away from the store, or taking your dog on a longer-than-usual walk.

don't worry (nan kuru nai sa; なん くる ない さ or 難来る無いさ)

The Okinawans appreciate the value of a strong mind. I have been practicing meditation for eight years now, and with each session, it becomes a little bit easier. I like to follow a guided meditation created by Deepak Chopra. Yes, some mornings I'm too committed to deadlines to meditate, but on these days, I make a promise to myself to save ten to thirty minutes of my day to do something for me.

Meditation is proven to lower stress levels; it helps to calm the mind and body, it alleviates anxiety and nervousness, and it helps to clear out the mental noise. Meditation also may help to slow the aging process. Best of all, anyone can do it, it's free, and it's simple to learn.

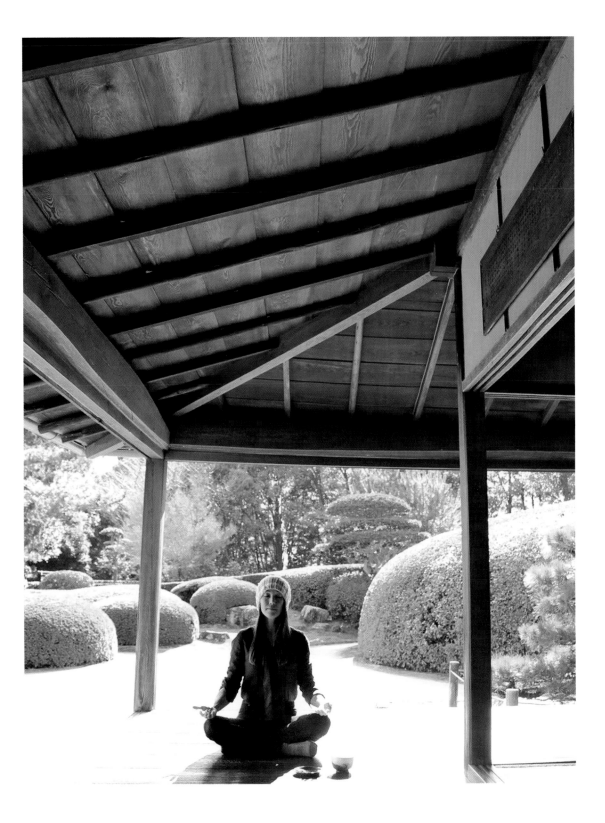

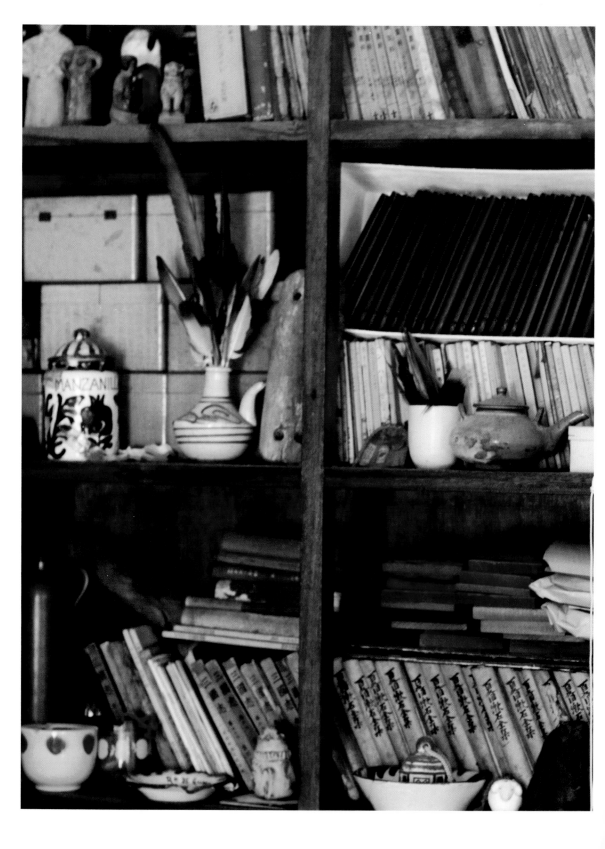

ganbatte

頑張って, がんばって

always do
your best

My Jiichan's artwork space was virtually left untouched. He was a true master with his Impressionist paintings, spreading his love of culture and travel through his work.

SOMEONE ONCE TOLD ME THAT HARD WORK DOES NOT GO UNNOTICED. I like to keep this in mind as I practice ganbatte, always doing my best.

Early in my career, I did a lot of comparing myself to others. Like many young people, I couldn't help but feel like everyone else was enjoying the ultimate success, and I didn't understand why my time wasn't revealing itself. In my twenties, I expected success to happen in an instant.

One example sticks out in my mind. At the time, I was twenty-five, young and hungry. I had the honor of working with one of the most talented book editors in the industry. Still, I was caught up in comparisons. I'll never forget the analogy she used with me about success, as I struggled (and, dude, did I struggle!) with finding peace in my heart regarding all I didn't yet have. As I sat at her desk side, she looked me in the eyes and said, "Candice, you have to think about success as a pan of pork chops. When you have one pork chop in the pan, it gets all dried up, but when you cook a few pork chops in the pan, together, they begin to keep each other moist and happy, and they come out perfect. There's enough room in the pan for everyone's success." I've never forgotten how hearing this made me feel.

It took me another decade of hard work, long hours, and many unpaid jobs to learn to be a better writer, manage my small business, and eventually be a better boss. But it is a continuous process, and I work on improving myself every day. Eventually, I learned to make peace with my own pace, my own trajectory. I didn't need to be at the top, but it was steadily building.

With time, age, experience, and hard work came opportunity.

I was raised to always do my best, and my dad is a remarkable example of ganbatte. He came to the U.S. on a boat from Poland when he was twelve years old. He learned English quickly (though it didn't come easily), and worked hard. Dad and his siblings made the very best of the opportunities they were given. My dad proudly served in the U.S. Navy as an electrician and my uncle John proudly served as a US Air Force Master Sergeant and, after, an Air National Guard Fire Department Captain.

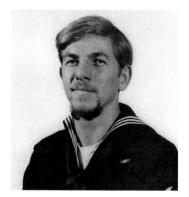

Dad came to the U.S. from Poland when he was just twelve. He worked so hard to later become successful on his own. When he met my mom, he was a young U.S. Navy sailor stationed in Japan. He said that "life was just better" with her. They are still best friends.

When I was growing up, my dad worked as a nuclear auditor, where he was responsible for overseeing and securing a nuclear power plant all day and night. In his career, it was incredibly necessary for him to be precise and accurate.

Mom was much the same in her own ways. The house was always spotless and in order. She threw the best birthday parties, she baked each of our cakes from scratch, and cooked every meal from scratch every day, in addition to her work as a school teacher. She always did her best. I would expect nothing less from her.

Anyone close to me will also tell you that my mother is my everything. Her words and her essence

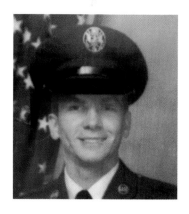

Uncle John dedicated his entire career to the service.

are my heart's anthem. I think of her on my toughest days. I thought of her in the kitchen when I was working on the line getting my arms burnt with tongs and coming home smelling like tempura. I kept her in the back of my mind when I got yelled at by my chef in the back alley beside the Dumpsters. I thought of her while writing at my desk in Brooklyn, barely making rent. I thought of her while I was working until 2:00 a.m., researching; fact checking; editing photos, layouts, recipes, and manuscripts.

I thought of Mom before walking on every set with my heels, in styled hair and makeup. I challenged myself to be impeccable with my reputation. After all, my mom was on the other side of the tube watching, and what would she think? I wanted to make her proud by doing my very best.

embrace the struggle

While kintsugi teaches us that there is beauty in the struggle, ganbatte says there is also beauty in the effort. Yes, the term *ganbatte* means that you must always give your best, but it also means that if you always do your best, that is good enough. You needn't be too hard on yourself, or expect perfection. You don't have to *be* the best, you just have to do *your* best.

To me, ganbatte is about always doing your best, but never seeing a ceiling to your capacity to do great work. I like to think of Martha Stewart as an example of this. I highly doubt she's ever found herself sitting at home saying, "Great job, Martha. You are now done. Congratulations."

In our everyday lives, how can we incorporate ganbatte? Here are a few ideas:

prepare: Preparation is huge. If you prepare a tremendous amount—for whatever is coming up—you'll be able to do your best. While preparation is specific to your situation, there are some things you should always do. Make sure to get plenty of rest. If that means no drinking caffeine that day, or putting your devices away and cutting the lights out early, do it. Condition your mind to stay calm throughout preparation, as it will help you to focus. You don't have to say yes to everything. When times are busy, don't overcommit. Before an important time or event, nourish yourself properly, drink plenty of water, and eat fresh foods. Staying away from alcohol is also a smart choice. When you feel your best, you do better work.

It is a Japanese custom to bring a gift to meetings. Part of my practice is to prepare a gift whenever I have a meeting. It can be something small, like homemade cookies, chocolate treats, or matcha tea. This small gesture goes a long way in letting people know that you think they are genuinely special and your relationship with them is important.

The other side of preparation is research. Growing up, I remember always watching my mother prepare her lesson plans. Although she has taught a similar Japanese language curriculum each year (for over forty years!), she still always prepares. The day before each class, she thinks about the next lesson, reviews the material, and studies. As a little girl, I'd hide behind her desk and watch her with glittering eyes. (She still doesn't know that I watched her.) Take a page from my mom and study up. If you're going to a job interview, research everything you can about the company and the people you'll be meeting with. Trust me, people love hearing that you researched up on them—it can only do you good.

Last but not least, practice. If you're giving a speech or presentation, practice, practice, practice. My dad is not naturally comfortable with public speaking, but I remember watching him practice giving speeches in our living room when I was a kid. Good preparation makes you fearless. You'll feel comfortable with the material before you step into the ring, and you will feel like you're up for anything.

give it your all: Time is limited. This is your one life, and some opportunities only come around once. Prepare for that job interview, that lunch date, that presentation—and then bring your absolute best self. If you want to truly achieve in your career, if you want to play at the top, you're going to have to give it your best. You get what you give.

be on time: Being punctual is polite, and it's also a favor you do for yourself. If you're rushing to make it to that important event on time, it's going to add stress and panic at a moment when what you really need is to be getting into your element. Being on time is often about planning ahead. Give yourself more time than you think you need to account for unforeseen circumstances, like traffic jams and train delays.

be yourself: Come as you are. Your strengths and talents make you different from other people. Growing up, my sister was an amazing dancer, but I could kick a ball. I was good at all the tomboy things, she was great at all the arty things. And later in life, we almost traded places. Jen is now a bike mechanic and writer, and I am a chef and writer. Everyone's gifts are very different, so your best will look different than other people's best. The way to ensure it is really *your* best is to keep it true to you.

wish others the best: Like so many things in life, ganbatte is also a reciprocal practice. When someone is about to go up for a big exam, speaking
event, job interview, meeting, wedding (really anything!), wish them the
best of luck and *mean it*. When you genuinely start to support the success
of others, it will come back to you!

At this point in my life, I believe in the reciprocal power of ganbatte
more than ever. That means putting your energy into supporting others, wishing them true success and showing up for them, being full of
light and love and sincere happiness. Life is not a competition. There is
enough room for everyone at the top, and no one can make it there without the honest support of others. But most of all, you must be true to
your work and wishes and mean what you say, practice what you believe,
and send sincere love, light, and energy their way, with a whole, honest
heart. *Ganbatte ne!*

be honest: My mother told me, "Always be honest; it will keep you out of
a lot of trouble." In Japanese culture, children are raised to believe that if
they are honest, they will be greatly rewarded. (In Japanese folktales, an
abundance of food and gold is given to characters that always do the right
thing.) My parents were always honest with Jenni and me, and with each
other. Honesty means embracing the truth with everyone—yourself and
others. Honesty shows you are real, you are doing your best, and you're
true to your core beliefs. Honesty allows people to trust you, and it inspires them to share their truth, too. If you want to be trusted, be honest.

Honesty is a trait that I have observed in each of the people I admire
most: Brené Brown, Marie Kondo, Oprah Winfrey, Marianne Williamson,

Melody Beattie, and Don Miguel Ruiz. Their work is what inspires me to come out of my shell and share my story. Honesty is apparent; it shows in your golden cracks. Each one is a symbol of bravery, and you should be proud to show it and to share it with others.

Olympic athletes are a great example of ganbatte in action. They devote their entire lives to playing their best game. They prepare, they practice, they take good care of themselves to ensure their performance is the very best it can be, and then they embrace their one shot and bring their all. That's *real* ganbatte. When we watch them, we feel inspired and naturally wish them our best. Use them as a guiding example of people who incorporate this practice into every part of their lives. Elite athletes show us how great they are—they do not need to tell us.

Ganbatte also means giving your best in your personal and private practices, not just in times where everyone is watching you. Ganbatte when you are writing an e-mail, ganbatte when you are cooking dinner, ganbatte when you are at home with your family. Take the lead from Japanese parents and do your best when you are setting an example for your children each day. Do your best when the world is watching, then do your best when nobody is watching.

Awards and prizes can feel good, and it's nice to be recognized for a significant achievement. But outside approval is by no means a measurement of or a testament to who you are. The true reward is feeling like you are making a difference in the world around you.

If you begin to practice ganbatte in your life, you will not only feel better, but also provide inspiration for others. Your efforts will reap rewards, and you will feel closer to your life's purpose. When you do your best from a place of love and sincerity, the whole world benefits.

kaizen—
continuously improving to the next level

While ganbatte can inspire you to bring your very best, the concept of *kaizen* encourages you to continuously improve. Kaizen says that while you may try your best, you will never reach your full potential. No matter how hard you try, you will always be improving yourself, improving your work, and improving the conditions of your life. Rather than being defeated by this, you can *always* strive to be better. All of us are constantly learning, growing, and improving as we go along. In Japan, kaizen is used predominantly in the business world, though the idea is something you are taught from the time you are a young child. As my father says, "Never be satisfied." Only then will you be able to reach ever higher.

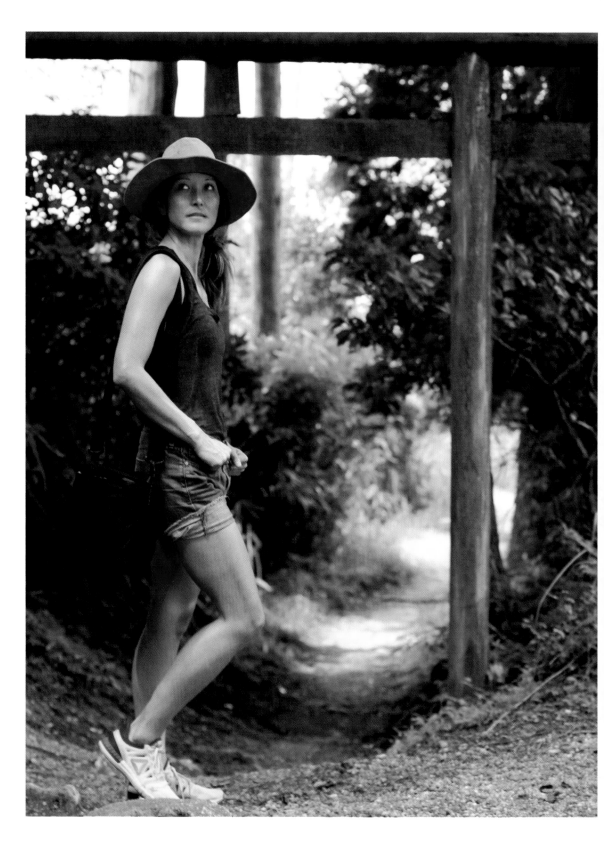

7

shikata ga nai

仕方が無い,

しかたがない

it cannot

be helped

Forest bathing in the mountains of Kōyasan is a form of letting go . . . practicing *shikata ga nai.*

Shikata ga nai, also known as *Shō ga nai*, しょうがない, is derived from the formal saying: "Don't keep complaining, move on from it."

One of the main reasons my Okinawan friend Hiromi-san says Okinawan women live so long? A little concept known as shikata ga nai, which means, "it cannot be helped." While I was in Okinawa, Hiromi-san explained to me that Japanese women "don't care so much" about the small things because they "have too many things to do."

At its essence, shikata ga nai (or shō ga nai) really means letting go. It means accepting what you cannot change and doing your best to let it roll off your back. It encourages you to take a step back from the drama in your life and remind yourself, "This won't matter in five years, or five months (or in some cases, even five weeks), so I'm not going to give it more than five minutes." And then wash your hands of it.

The trees in autumn are a good example of shikata ga nai in nature. The seasons are changing; it cannot be helped. As the leaves fall, the trees show us an example of letting go.

Taking a page from Okinawan women, when you encounter something that cannot be changed (like a disagreement with a stubborn person, or even inclement weather), don't dwell on it. "Shō ga nai," let it go, it cannot be helped. What you can change is the power and direction of your whole life, just by changing your mind-set. Take a deep breath. Ease up. Let it go.

When you have an argument or a falling-out with a friend, where no matter how hard you try, you just can't see eye to eye, it can be a relief to just let it go. Some things cannot be helped. It might take the form of a job you didn't get, a date that didn't go well, or a cancelled flight. You aren't going to be able to change certain circumstances, and you aren't going to be able change the way some people feel.

When you find yourself confronted with a situation that can't be helped, it can be tempting to torture yourself, wondering what went wrong, blaming yourself, or else trying to fix something or make something work. Dwelling or ruminating on the past prevents healing and dims your light. This kind of self-torture is a dishonorable and disrespectful thing to do to yourself. More often than not, when something cannot be helped, it is a sign that it was truly not meant to be. It doesn't matter—shikata ga nai!

If you're currently in that place, it might be time to do the harder thing by walking away. When you let go of something not meant for you, you will find relief. You will feel peace. You may not find it instantaneously. Sometimes you do see the value by just stepping away, and sometimes it takes longer to gain perspective. When you're in the midst of a tough situation, it can feel like you're in the middle of the forest, and all you can see is the trees. (Or like you're in the middle of the city, and all you can see is buildings.) But by walking away, you're taking yourself out of the situation and putting yourself in a new setting. Before you know it, you'll have a new vantage point and be able to see the entire landscape. Shikata ga nai, let it go.

family matters

For decades I watched my mother handle difficult times with such grace, honor, and dignity. She never complained about anything.

I can only imagine how hard it was for her to raise two American girls as a Japanese immigrant, but my mom did it. She took pride in being a mom, and would give Jenni and me extra schoolwork if there was a subject where we needed improvement. She always stayed true to what she believed in, and loyal to her ancestry. That meant remaining calm, truthful, and patient. She continued to show me how to be strong, how to study, how to work with integrity, how to be punctual, how to be the best I could possibly be. She rarely spoke ill of others, and did not gossip, even when things weren't going her way. And she always maintained her sense of humor (my mom is by far the funniest person in our family, she just doesn't know it).

Of course, we weren't perfect. Like any family, we had fights, struggles, and family meetings. I was a bad teenager who hung out with the wrong kids and argued with the other members of my family. They'd probably tell you that's an understatement. (I'm sorry, Mom and Dad! I will make it up to you!) My parents didn't always know how to handle my insubordination. Over the years, my family and I have communicated and miss-communicated. But sometimes we found the best answer was simply shō ga nai, just letting something go. Ultimately, I'm grateful for the struggles and setbacks we shared together, as they have made us all into who we are today. Without these times of turmoil and change, the ups and downs, we would not be able to learn and grow or enrich our lives. The struggles will become your story. And that's the beauty of kintsugi. Your cracks can become the most beautiful part of you.

roll with the punches

Shikata ga nai is all about rolling with the punches, allowing your sails to go in the direction of the wind. If you open your arms, your mind, your dreams, your sails to the wind, and you work in sync with all that life brings you, you will find that all things just get a little easier. It's not always the strongest and smartest who go the furthest; it is often those who can adapt.

Adaptation is a Japanese art. The next time you are going through a not-so-great situation I urge you to remember the Japanese way: stay calm, stay resilient, breathe, and adapt to the course.

After the 2016 election, my sister and I were devastated. My dad wrote a very thoughtful letter to us in which he said not to sweat the small stuff. He told us that a politician did not need to infiltrate our everyday lives. He said that others will be president—including a woman—and that we can continue to do good things for others and to enjoy ourselves. My dad is not a man of many words, so when he speaks, you really listen. His words of shikata ga nai meant a lot to me.

When something external goes wrong, remember: Don't take anything personally. It's a pretty safe bet that it's not about you.

Practicing shikata ga nai can take many forms in your daily life. Walking is one of the main reasons the Japanese maintain their cool and live such long lives, so the next time you're struggling, walk it off. For me, a very peaceful and simple meditation each morning has allowed me to be a calmer, more resilient, and more chill person. Meditation helps me to nip anxiety in the bud. Practicing yoga with like-minded friends has strengthened my spirit and made me a more peaceful person. Find your personal practice that helps you stay calm and centered.

Also, self-knowledge is power. The next time you're put in a high-stress situation, observe your behavior! Do you react right away? Do you reach for something healthy or unhealthy? Picking up a glass of wine, a beer, or a cocktail is easy. If we can do the harder thing and learn to better discipline ourselves by working on our mental focus, clarity, and bodily health in times of distress, imagine how much stronger (both mentally and physically) we will become.

Here are some more ways you can practice shikata ga nai:

meditate: As I mentioned, my morning meditation practice does wonders for curbing my anxiety and helping me to be more open and accepting of what I cannot help. To begin, you can meditate by sitting quietly in your home or in nature. You can find a mediation center or a group meditation practice. You can also try a guided recording or a meditation app, like Headspace.

breathe deeply: Deep breathing—especially through the nose—can help you feel grounded and take you back to reality. As you breathe deeply, scan your body and notice whether you are holding on to any tension. Are you clenching your jaw or furrowing your eyebrows? Deep breathing has been shown to have an immediate effect on blood pH, which lowers your blood pressure and calms your entire body. Plus, when you make it a regular practice, deep breathing benefits the mind, heart, digestion, and immune system.

immerse yourself: Whether it's your work, reading a good book, a hobby, traveling, or an interest that makes you feel better, choose to immerse yourself in something productive instead of dwelling or ruminating on negative thoughts. Fresh ideas, new content, and work you care about will help carry your mind to a better place.

pick yourself up: I like to get fresh flowers for myself, whether at the grocery store or the corner market. It really brightens up my space and makes me happy! Whether it's a fresh bouquet or something else—a candle, a favorite treat, a warm bath—give yourself the things you need to feel good.

tune in: Sound can be an incredible mood booster. Each day, I listen to music that makes me feel good or try a podcast that makes me feel inspired and helps me learn new things. There are so many options out there, on every topic imaginable.

always be learning: Stay curious. Read things. Talk to people. Take classes. The more you know, the more empowered and aware you become.

stop comparing: Comparing your life to the lives of others is always a self-defeating practice. The only person you should ever compare yourself to is . . . you. If you find yourself playing the comparison game, look away from the news or social media, and engage more in real life. Take some alone time. Make a note of all the things you love and the things you do well. Grant yourself that serenity.

tend to your own garden: This means, get in touch with your place in the natural world, and care for yourself as you would a seedling. Nourish, hydrate, get sun. If you're busy with life's demands, this doesn't have to mean you take a whole day or night in your PJs. But do find a pocket of me-time. Prioritize yourself as number one.

healing objects: It helps to have some symbolic reminders to stay the course. I love my healing stones and crystals, especially my rose quartz, to help bring love into my life. Crystals are very accessible, and having them around makes me feel better. I also like my mala beads (a traditional meditation necklace with 108 beads), which I used to help myself feel grounded while I was going through a difficult time. You can use them as a tool during meditation, but I would hold them before bed and they would make me feel better. Maybe crystals aren't your thing, and that's okay. Find something—a quote, an image, a symbolic item from your family—that resonates with you.

change your perspective: Getting a change of scenery can do wonders for taking yourself out of an unfixable situation and seeing it from a new perspective. This doesn't have to mean a trip or vacation—although it could. You can get a new perspective by walking to a part of town you don't normally go to, driving a different route, visiting someone you haven't seen in a while, or watching a documentary.

go hiking/forest bathing: While we're on the topic of taking in the scenery, spending time in nature is a fresh way to practice shikata ga nai. In Japan, the practice of walking slowly through the woods, taking time to contemplate, is known as forest bathing (*shinrin yoku*). Breathing fresh oxygen into your body, inhaling the natural oils released from the trees, and being able to touch, smell, and see something outside of your situation will help to open up a lot of channels that may have been closed off to you. It will open your mind to looking at things from a different vantage point. Take yourself out of your element.

hang with supportive friends: Everybody needs friends who uplift them. Assess who makes you feel good, and look to those people for support when you're grappling with a situation that cannot be helped.

Remember, shikata ga nai is not an easy practice, and it's something that you will need to work on continuously. After all, you cannot ask the universe to stop giving you problems. Everyone has them. But you can learn how to roll with the punches, and if you do the work, then over time, I promise it will feel easier.

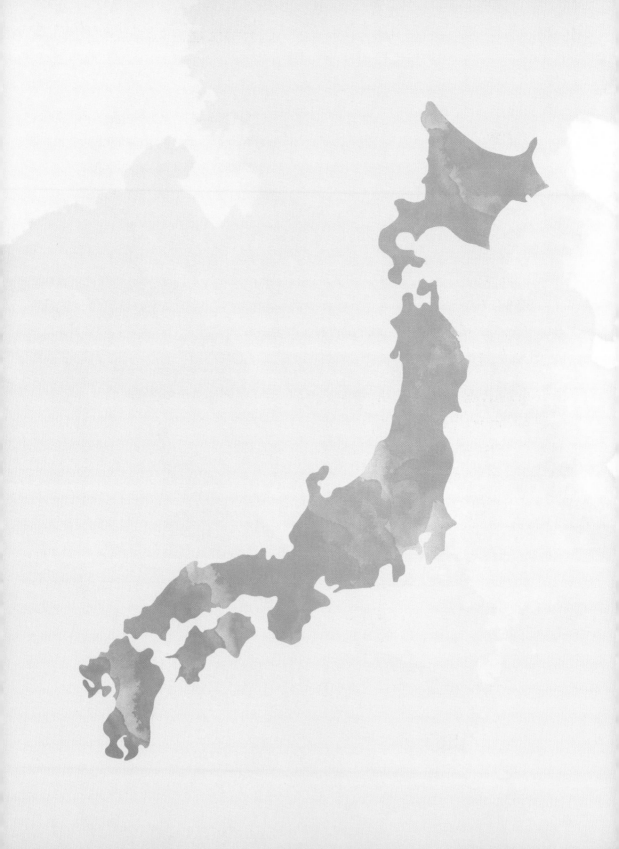

IV

heart
kokoro
ハート, 心, こころ

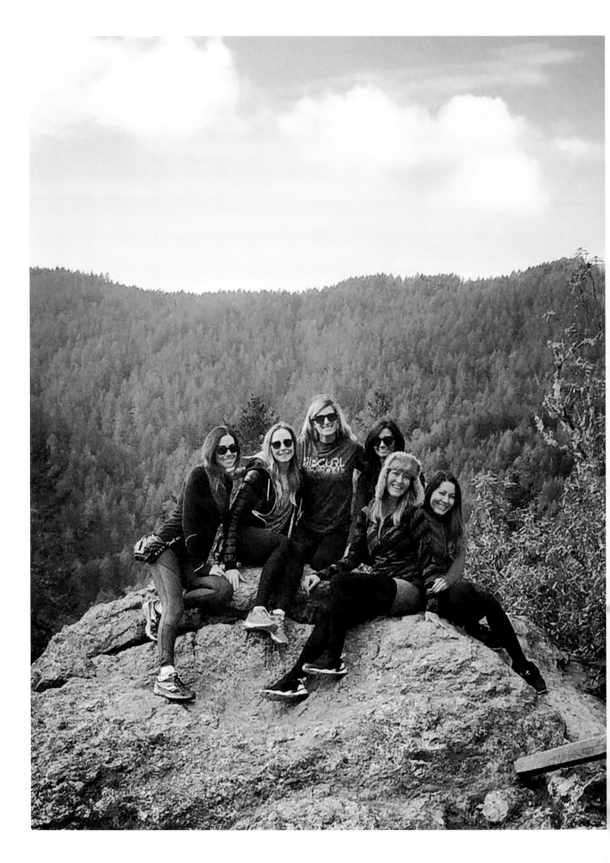

8

yuimaru

ゆいまーる

inner circle

of people

My best friends took me hiking (forest bathing) during a time when I needed healing. My forever yuimaru.

THE OKINAWAN CULTURE USES THE TERM *YUIMARU*, WHICH TRANSLATES TO "THE CIRCLE OF THE PEOPLE." Yuimaru is a concept that celebrates the value of togetherness. It teaches us that our social networks, particularly our inner circle of close friends, heal us and help strengthen and nourish our entire community.

Yuimaru was another lesson I witnessed firsthand. Okinawa is a diverse, multicultural island, including many people from Japan and the United States. In such a mixed population, the concept of yuimaru feels very present. Everywhere I went, there was a feeling of unity, compassion, and sincerity.

I observed how my Okinawan friends supported their neighborhood restaurants, pottery shops, musical performances, and dancing events. There is a strong embrace of the local community. In my own life, I've always felt it's better to have close friends, family, and a community you can grow strong and loyal with than to have a ton of casual friends or acquaintances.

In life, we will inevitably go through tough times. It's important to be mindful that we all need to rely on one another in order to survive. Sharing our successes amplifies them. Sharing our struggles makes them easier to endure. You're not going to be able to make it alone. That's why we are all here on this one big, crazy planet together. Whatever it is you are trying to accomplish, it helps to lean on your yuimaru.

It will take your tribe, your posse, your squad, your team. You may stumble—in fact, you may fall right on your face (as I have many times), and that's okay. Supported by your inner circle, you will be able to get up gracefully and with resilience and back on your two feet.

being vulnerable

Everyone is vulnerable, whether they want to admit it or not. Vulnerability is not a sign of weakness; being vulnerable is actually a sign of strength. As we learn throughout our times of trauma and pain, our struggles and setbacks, vulnerability can be difficult, but ultimately we will be okay.

Ironically, I've discovered that the ability to be present and vulnerable with others begins with being alone. I need my alone time to recharge. When I spend time alone, I become more comfortable with myself, so that when I am with others, I'm more able to be open.

When I traveled to Japan on my own six years ago, I had a tremendous amount of healing to do, and I wanted to take the time to focus on self-care so I could heal properly. It was tough to be so open with my emotions, but I realized that being vulnerable is also an immense opportunity to learn valuable lessons, and to get clear on the things that you want and need out of life.

I spent that year surrounding myself with a community of only the most supportive and engaged people, and I noticed a shift begin to happen in my life.

I actually liked who I was. I found my work more meaningful. And I wanted to focus on making a deep impact on the lives of others. I learned to love myself and take care of myself the way I would a best friend.

Perhaps that was the biggest shift of all: When I was alone, I was surprised to find that I could treat myself as if I were my own best friend. Traveling alone gave me the ability to be present. It was a remarkable and unexpected shift. After this realization, I was able to be a better friend, because I was truly present when I was with the people I loved. I began to speak with an open heart. I didn't hesitate to share my needs and my vulnerability.

The real work behind vulnerability, however, happens when you are open to being vulnerable with others. When I became more vulnerable, I took my mask off and let everyone in on my secrets. I became transparent and finally had the guts to share my story, to live in each moment, and to own it as if it were my last time to share.

Vulnerability is about being brave. It means being open and honest, and not afraid of judgment, rejection, or pain. When we are vulnerable, we can open our hearts to new ideas, new relationships, and new people! Once I began to open up, incredible people entered my life. Sometimes friendships and foundations actually begin to solidify when you are most broken open—as you embrace the broken places, it allows you to grow. Being vulnerable is the first step in this process.

make the commitment

On my last trip to Japan, my mom and I spent a couple of days in Tokyo viewing the cherry blossoms. One day, we met up for lunch with Mom's lifelong friends from her college days. In Japan, it's traditional to give one another gifts. (They don't have to be anything fabulous. The gifts usually take the form of a small token like a handkerchief, a teacup, or cookies.)

My heart was touched as each of Mom's friends gave me a gift. One even made me four of her cherished homemade Japanese recipes, which I will always remember.

As we sat at lunch, I interviewed them about their friendship. "How is it possible that Mom lives in California, and over the years, all of you have stayed in touch?" They said it was a lot of work and that it took commitment. They had to plan times to speak, and once a year they arrange to see one another. Keeping a friendship alive over the years is work, but it's definitely worth it.

embrace community

Community makes a positive impact and a lasting imprint on the human heart. Having a strong and centered community around you, whether through a church, book club, cooking class, yoga, art or meditation class, healing group, cycling club, recreational sport, whatever it may be, is important to your well-being. Building a strong sense of community improves your motivation, health, and happiness. Karyn Hall, PhD, explains that when you're part of a close-knit community, you're more cognizant of the fact that all people struggle and go through difficult times. Thus, there is comfort in knowing that you are not alone. Furthermore, researchers have found that people are happier when they are around others as opposed to being alone. Social support is a critical component of mental health and healthy aging.

This is Shizuko, my grandmother's best friend and neighbor for over sixty-five years. Throughout their lives, she and my grandmother relied on each other for friendship, laughter, loyalty, and company. Shizuko's parents taught her "Be good to your neighbor." And she was! Shizuko adored my Baachan and cherished their time together. I had the honor to speak with Shizuko while I was visiting Beppu just after my grandmother passed away. She shared with me the newfound appreciation she had for the friends in her life. Shizuko told me, "I was a very selfish person, up until my eighties." She never told her friends how much they meant to her, and never expressed her gratitude for having them in her life.

When Shizuko was in her eighties, many of her friends moved or passed away, and she began to feel alone—she was left with nobody. Once they were gone, she realized how much they truly mattered to her. "It wasn't until then that I realized being selfish wasn't the way I should be living my life," she said. "You can't live alone, you've got to thank your friends."

So at age eighty, Shizuko decided to make a change. She began to be more vulnerable. She opened up to those around her, she communicated more honestly, and she gave her heart fully. She has a regular gratitude practice and you can feel it in her warm and attentive presence. While in Beppu, I would see her at the market every day, where she would grab me by the hand and give me the warmest greeting. She always greeted others with a huge smile, and was all too happy to stop and chat. Even though many of her lifelong friends, my grandmother included, are no longer around, Shizuko continued to make new connections rather than keeping to herself.

Shizuko taught me the importance of valuing and appreciating friendships, new and old. Open up to them, make time for them, don't wait to tell the people you care about that you love them and are grateful for their presence. Start living with an open heart now. We only have so much time.

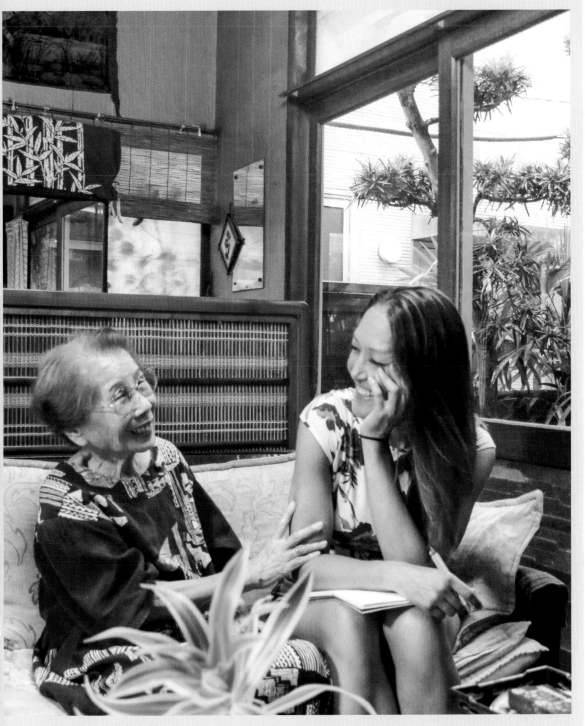

Shizuko, ninety-six, my grandmother's best friend for over sixty-five years, sharing with me her thoughts on a lifetime of honoring friendship.

show, don't tell

Just as kaizen teaches us to practice continuous improvement, we can apply the same idea to relationships, focusing much of our time on continuous support. That's what the circle is all about. Just as my friends and family are always there for me, I try hard to always be there for them.

Of course, actions are the true measure of the friendship you offer to others. If you want to be a good friend to someone, show them! For example, many of us are quick to connect over text or e-mail—we don't even talk to our friends anymore. Scheduling time to connect with someone over tea or a meal shows them that they are valuable to you. Spending time with and taking time for the people in your life matters—it is one of the ways you can express their value in your life. To love other people is to feel loved. And that, my love, is the truth.

Here are some other ways to practice friendship in action:

be thoughtful: Holidays and obvious occasions are great times to show people you love and care, but when you text someone out of the blue to tell them that you love them, that can feel more meaningful. Likewise, there is no expiration date on giving thanks. If you really enjoy something a friend gave you three years ago, tell them how much you still love it! If an old memory pops into your head, let them know you thought of them! I'll get messages every week from someone who made my recipes, and it truly makes my day. Everyone loves to know they are appreciated, no matter the day.

be present: Give others your attention. Are you on your phone the entire time you're at dinner? (Seriously, put your phone away, like, all the way away.) Are you listening intently to your friend's story? Human connection depends on attention. Sincerely ask people how they are and actually listen to their response.

share yourself: It's okay to share your true emotion, to show your vulnerable parts, to be real. Witnessing the deep parts of others brings people comfort, because it is only then that we see we are not alone. Don't be afraid of what others think, or feel that you have to put on a brave face. That may be true in certain circumstances, but when you are with your yuimaru, it's okay to fearlessly share what's really going on.

offer support: Use your talents to help a friend, even if it's just lending an ear. If you have a service you can offer, give it freely and happily to those who can benefit. The favor will come back around.

don't expect anything in return: Live and give without expectation. For those you truly love, there will be a natural exchange. But never offer your support because you're trying to get credit in the favor bank. It's pretty obvious when somebody is coming after you needing something in return. Your interactions with friends should be sincere, and come from a place of pure good intention, without any ulterior motives.

be proactive: Friendship is about offering support even when someone *doesn't* ask. It's checking in on a friend when you know they're waiting on news (good or bad) or have a big day coming up at work. It can also mean bringing hot soup to a friend who's sick at home, or picking up a few things at the grocery store for a friend with a new baby. It could be writing an encouraging note or e-mail for a friend who has a big interview or presentation coming up. Friendship is defined by actions, and it is also defined by not having to ask for what you need. Your true friends know just what you need and when, and they are happy to offer their support.

I know who my true circle of friends is—my yuimaru, my posse, my squad—because they are the first ones to step up to the plate in tough times. They're the girlfriends who squeeze in a yoga class with me even though their schedule is jam-packed, who come over to hold my hand through a breakup, who sincerely want to come out to toast and celebrate my birthday or a big accomplishment. They are happy for my successes, as I am sincerely over-the-moon happy for theirs. They are the safety net that continues to catch me and to lift me up, higher and higher. When you're being true to yourself, you know that your circle is there around you for the right reasons—the real you.

Tokyo, Japan: My mom and her best friends from university. They studied to be teachers together in Tokyo, decades ago, and are an example of a long-term yuimaru.

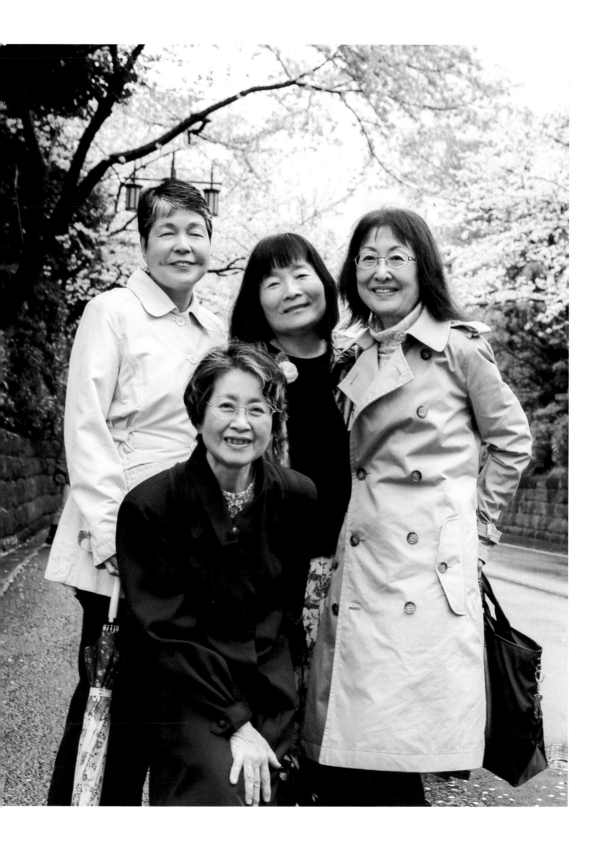

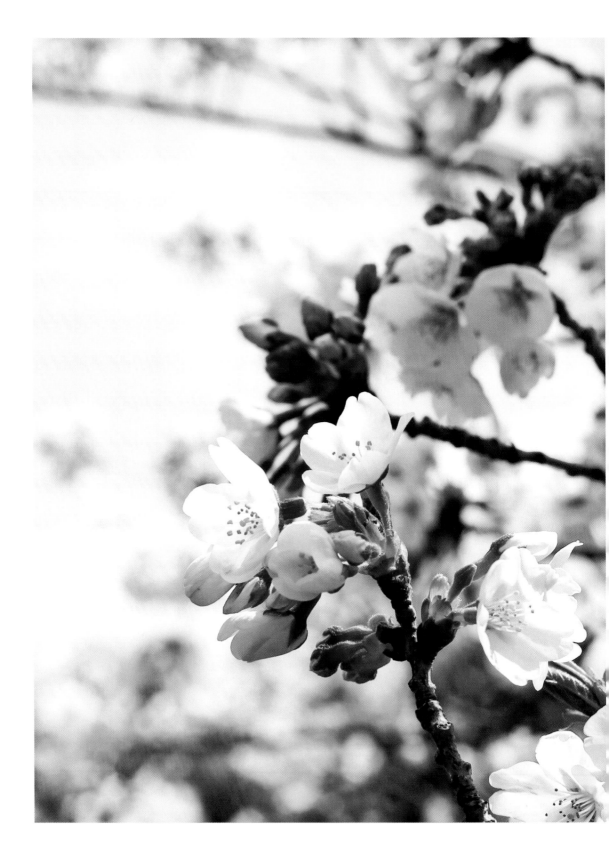

9

kansha

感謝, かんしゃ

gratitude

| Kamakura, Japan.

ONE OF THE MOST IMPORTANT CONCEPTS IN YOUR WELLNESS PRACTICE—THE ONE THAT SUPPORTS ALL THE OTHERS—IS THE JAPANESE PHILOSOPHY KNOWN AS *KANSHA*. At its heart, *kansha* means "cultivating gratitude." This includes gratitude for the gifts you've been given, for this moment, and for everything in this one lifetime.

My parents are from two very different cultures and religions, but, despite their different upbringings, both are rooted in deep and sincere gratitude. They openly expressed their gratitude for what we had, and shared their appreciation with my sister and me.

The beginning of their relationship (what would become a lifetime of love) started in a place of peace: the Great Buddha at Kamakura, a coastal city just south of Tokyo.

The Japanese have a tradition of telling folktales to their children in order to pass on the beauty and tradition of kansha. There are two that really stand out: *Tsuru no Ongaeshi* ("The Grateful Crane"), and *Kasa Jizō* ("Umbrella Statue"). Both stories focus on teaching children that if you're a good person who practices gratitude, you'll be rewarded. They also share traditional and deep-rooted values and morals with their little ones through manga (Japanese comics) and Japanese animation.

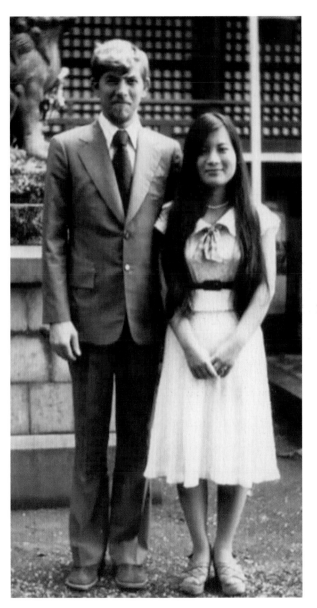

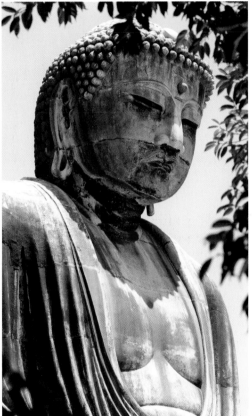

LEFT: Mom and Dad, Beppu, Japan, 1973: I asked what drew them together, although they were so different. They replied similarly, "We wanted to see the world together."

RIGHT: Kamakura, Japan: This is a sacred place for the Japanese, a place the samurai once called their capital. This temple marks the spot where our family kansha began when my parents met there in the seventies.

kawaii: major cuteness

Speaking of animation, Japanese culture is extremely unique in its appreciation for cute things. Just as wabi-sabi teaches us to see beauty in the imperfect, *kawaii* teaches us to find humor and happiness in cuteness. Hello Kitty, Mario and Luigi, Doraemon, Pokémon, Rilakkuma . . . and emoji are all examples of this. Happiness inspires gratitude, as it is a celebration of living. I urge you to look for the fun and humor around you. In Japanese culture, we appreciate spreading kawaii, which inspires lightness.

In Japan there is a saying, *ongaeshi,* which translates to "always return the favor." My entire life I watched my mother and father devote much of their free time outside of work to volunteering in our community, and they've kept up with it to this day. My mom volunteers at our local Japanese school, where she helps to raise funds for Japanese cultural education and the preservation of Japanese tradition in our community. Mom also donates to humane animal organizations every year. Every week, my dad volunteers at a charity thrift store, at my former high school, and at the Boys and Girls Club. When I asked him why he chooses to spend so much of his time volunteering, he said, "It's satisfying to help others and to give back to the community." It seems so obvious on the surface, and yet so few of us make the time to actually do it. But giving back is a part of practicing kansha. By giving back, we expand our perspective on what we have, and what we can give to others.

Here are some ways to actively practice gratitude:

practice patience: Kansha takes practice. You can't always see it clearly, and it can be difficult to feel grateful when the truth is life is hard sometimes. It wasn't until I became more confident in myself that I started to feel and understand sincere gratitude.

I didn't always understand kansha. Part of growing up means letting go of your sense of self-importance, feeling more grace, having more empathy and compassion. We are like stones that get washed up on the shore. They've been tossed through so many waves that they've become smooth and polished, but it takes a lot of waves before they take on that shape. Be patient; gratitude grows with time.

"A smile radiates from the heart."
—JAPANESE PROVERB

give your gratitude as a handwritten card or a smile: Showing gratitude can be simple. I believe a handwritten thank-you card is still one of the greatest joys to open. You can be certain it will make the recipient smile because they know the time and effort that went into that personal note. Little things add up—and when you make others happy, you are making yourself happy. So ditch the premade thank-you cards and let your own version of kansha shine!

As a thank-you, I love to visit the flower district in New York City and select a fresh, gorgeous assortment of flowers. I bring them home and set up mason jars. Then I'll arrange flowers in each one for a friend, and attach a simple thank-you note to each one. I keep their individual tastes and preferences in mind, making a gift I know they'll love. As a final touch, I always hand deliver them to the people in my life who I want to thank. It's a way to make others smile and to show my sincere appreciation.

But of course, you don't have to do what I do! There are lots of ways to express your gratitude. Bake some cookies, write some letters, frame a picture of you and your friends together; you'll be having fun and spreading more kansha into the world.

develop gratitude for your character: When you feel you have nothing to offer, remember you always have your character.

In my early twenties, I went through a period of feeling lost. I remember calling my parents with my head down to say, "I'm really sorry, but I need your help." Dad and I packed up my things, loaded them into a U-Haul, and moved me back to my parents' house, without a plan.

I had never felt so low, and wondered if things would ever get better. Instead of feeling sorry for myself, my dad encouraged me to start filling my résumé with volunteer and community work. He told me that being of service to others would help me to appreciate my own path.

Soon after, I attended an event at my local bookstore for a book written by two teachers. The book detailed the number of people in both our community and the nation who were forced to live on food stamps. After the event, I met a few women who invited me to work at a local breadline in Encinitas, California, where I began to help out two days a week. My dad was right; it felt good to give back and connect with those in need in my community. To go from the mounds of food and drink that came along with my former life to the food bank, where so many people had to wait in line for something to feed their families, was eye-opening. That gap was wide and understanding it was a very powerful moment for me.

That experience began to deepen my gratitude and my character. From where I stand, I am grateful for those past struggles and setbacks. I'm grateful for those times when my bank account was overdrawn, when I had no apartment or job.

I often think and reflect on these times as a reminder of how grateful I am now. I can now look back and wonder, had my life never fallen apart back then, would I be who I am today? Probably not. That's kintsugi, the restoring of one's life.

Being of service is an ongoing part of my gratitude practice. Now much of my charitable work is focused on hunger and better nutrition in my community. Whatever cause speaks to you, I encourage you to give back however you can. You may find, as I have, that it is an essential part of being your community.

togetherness (issho! 一緒 いっしよ!): In Japanese culture, meals are a sacred time for a family to sit down and eat in each other's company. *Issho* means "together." It can also mean "one place, same time." Growing up, my dad always said it to my mom (like when they were going to Costco) as a term of endearment.

Before each meal, it is customary to say *Itadakimasu*, which pays gratitude to every part of the meal, and every person who was involved at any point with the creation of the meal. We would thank our parents (typically we would thank Mom for cooking the meal, and thank Dad for being a provider). At the end of each meal, you conclude by saying, *Gochisōsama deshita,* meaning the meal was delicious and sending thanks to the chef.

Growing up, it was rare for us to eat apart. Japanese families often travel together, as well. Each time I would travel to Japan, my mom and I would make daily trips to the market, to cook and eat together at Baachan's house. We felt very lucky when my Baachan and my Great-Auntie Takuko (her sister) joined us.

The older I've grown, the more I've come to value "togetherness," especially with my sister, my mom, my dad, and my best friends.

cultivate sincerity: When I think about Japanese culture, there is one word that always comes to mind: sincere. I talked about the importance of sincerity in wishing someone *ki o tsukete,* but it extends to all parts of life. To me, sincerity means connecting with someone in the most authentic way, where your true self acknowledges his or her true self. It is about communicating with honesty, about acting in accordance with your beliefs, about having the other person's best interests in mind because you truly care. It is having moral integrity.

When we practice kansha, we are opening our hearts, allowing ourselves to feel gratitude, and sparking something beautiful. But the key ingredient to kansha is sincerity—putting your heart behind everything you say and do. Be sincere when you pay a compliment to a coworker about the presentation they made. See how you feel inside when you sincerely tell your girlfriend you haven't seen in a month how glowing and gorgeous she looks!

Think about your work: Is it meaningful? Do you love to tell others about it? Does it evoke emotion, change? Does it create time and space for you to be sincere? When you say good morning to your work colleagues, how sincere are you in your delivery? Is it possible that you could create some changes in your daily life to evoke more sincerity?

Try not to practice false gratitude—if you don't feel it, don't say it. Everyone wants to feel loved, needed, and part of a community. You have the power, the capacity, the life, and the breath to be this person in everyone's lives. But in order to do so, you have to be sincere. Be positive, be complimentary, be the sunshine in people's lives, and, before you know it, that light will shine back onto you.

Remember, you cannot simply pick up sincerity at the corner market, nor can you master it in a week. It takes work, inward searching, and struggle to give you the experience that allows you to authentically relate to others. This is another way the cracks that become part of us throughout our lives are really a gift—kintsugi is life experience, and life experience allows us to have deeper, more meaningful empathy for one another.

practice gratitude for the past: In Japanese culture, it's customary to respect your elders, and part of this practice is rooted in gratitude. Honoring your elders includes spending time with them, listening to their stories, and learning from them. Wisdom from our ancestors is one of the best gifts we can receive.

Instead of trying to write a new wellness theory, we can learn from our wise ancestors who are all too happy to hand it down to us. Wellness isn't found in supplements or diets. Wellness isn't something you can buy. True wellness can be found by studying our past and our traditions. I wish that Western culture looked at our elders in a special light, the way I observed people in Japan do. We must learn to accept their gifts with gratitude.

Whenever people ask me the question "If you could invite anyone to dinner, who would it be?" I always say my grandparents. I wish I could have one meal with both my Japanese and Polish grandparents. I was so young when they were with us, and there was a language barrier. We would laugh and cook together, but I never got to ask them the questions I would ask them now, about their lives growing up, about Poland and Japan during the war, about the stories that held meaning for them in their lives. If you are lucky enough to have elders in your life, do not take them for granted. Instead, practice kansha, and be thankful for the wisdom they can offer.

I'll never forget my seventy-plus-year-old guide Noda-san, who took me hiking on the beautiful island of Shikoku. (You can meet Noda-san and read more about the Shikoku pilgrimage on page 268.) She had visited all eighty-eight temples on the long and arduous pilgrimage more than twenty-six times. I asked her how she felt about the rigors of her job, and she just looked at me with her deep, sincere eyes and told me, "Candice, I love my job, and I am so proud of what I do." This is not uncommon in Japan. The people I met all had similar reactions to my question.

The couple I met and interviewed in the Noto Peninsula, the Maekawa family, have produced traditional *hoshigaki* or *korogaki* (dried persimmons) for decades, just as their parents and grandparents did. When we asked the husband, Mister Maekawa, who is in his eighties, if he was ready to retire, he just laughed and said, "No, I'm not ready to retire. When I am ready, I will pass this practice on to my [nearly sixty-year-old] son and he will take over the business." He was filled with gratitude for his lineage and his heritage, and took deep pride in his work.

Watching the older generation at work—the light in their eyes, their dedication to detail, perfection, and integrity—has a way of making you feel you should work harder. Many generations of Japanese people have chosen to dedicate their whole lives to their work, and they sincerely derive joy from a job well done. We must learn from this older generation, show our respect, pay homage to them, and pass along these traditions of sincerity, respect, and heart.

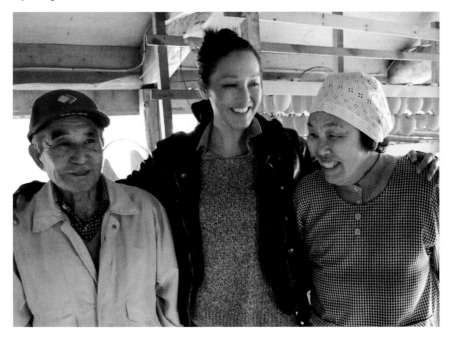

The Maekawa family shows us gratitude. Devotion to their work is a common prcatice among traditional Japanese.

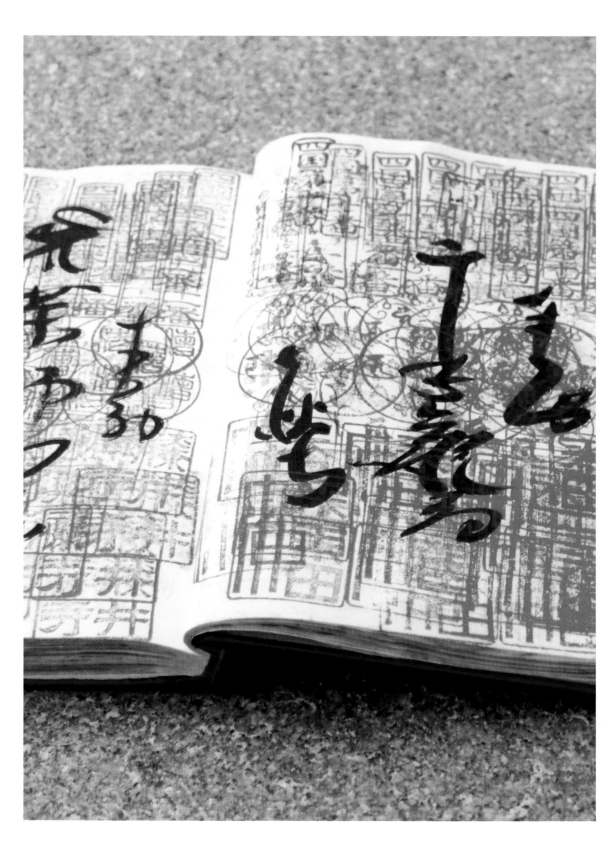

10

osettai

お接待,おせったい

be of service,

welcoming gifts.

Shikoku, Japan: My favorite guide, Noda-san, shares with me her incredibly valuable prayer book. Books like this are humbly preserved over a lifetime of pilgrimage.

THE LAST STOP ON MY MOST RECENT JAPANESE JOURNEY WAS SHIKOKU, THE SMALLEST OF JAPAN'S FOUR MAIN ISLANDS AND A SACRED PLACE TO WHICH THOUSANDS MAKE AN ANNUAL PILGRIMAGE. Known as the Ohenro pilgrimage, this eighty-eight-temple journey through the Shikoku Mountains is at the top of many Japanese people's bucket lists. The true pilgrimage consists of a visit to all eighty-eight temples, where a pilgrim will pray and have their prayer book stamped. Beyond that, however, there are no rules; simply showing up and starting to walk qualifies one as an Ohenro pilgrim. Traditionally, the pilgrimage is made on foot, which takes over fifty days. Some people (less than 5 percent) still do it this way, though most modern pilgrims make the trek by car or bus in less than a week.

Recently, following the popularity of the Camino de Santiago pilgrimage in Northern Spain, more Westerners have taken an interest in Shikoku's arduous trail. However, given the distances involved and the relative remoteness of the destination, one can still go several days along the journey without meeting another non-Japanese pilgrim, which is what I think makes it so cool.

Prayer books are important on the pilgrimage. These beautiful books are filled with many red-ink prints and are considered to be very valuable. As I started my pilgrimage, I met a few Shikoku residents, Yuka, Yuki, and our amazing guide, Noda-san. The locals are consistently warm and welcoming to foreign pilgrims, offering them small gifts and words of support along the way. My new friends were no exception. Since I had never been before, they invited me to join them and offered to be my guides. As we began to travel up the hills to our first temple, they first shared the term *osettai*. They told me the term is local to Shikoku and refers to the gifts pilgrims receive along their journey. In this case, the gifts aren't only material things, but also the warm welcome one receives, and the hospitality these traveling pilgrims encounter along their journey. They explained to me that even the sunshine on that particular day could be considered osettai, since it made our hiking conditions hospitable. Whenever the world gives you a day of sunshine, that is osettai. Allow yourself to bask in it, as gifts are to be enjoyed and appreciated.

The greatest takeaway from my journey was not a material souvenir, but a new spirit, rooted in the understanding of what it means to be a gracious host. My guides showed me that any form of hospitality counts as osettai. Hosting friends or family members is osettai. Helping a grandmother walk up the mountain—or even just across the street—counts as osettai because it is a gift to help ease someone's journey. Giving up your seat on the train counts as your daily osettai.

As Yuki-san explained, "Osettai also includes warm wishes sent to people, or that people send you. Maybe someone cannot go on the pilgrimage together with you, but they entrust you with their wishes, and thus go on the pilgrimage through their osettai." In your own life, simply praying for others to have a safe journey can be part of an osettai practice.

It was plain to see how osettai—gifts, invitations, warm welcomes—is so rooted in the way the people of Shikoku live. This beautiful spirit of generosity creates a feeling of warmth and joy whenever you are around them.

My time in Shikoku was transformative. This leg of my pilgrimage

k i n t s u g i
金継ぎ
w e l l n e s s

included only five temples, but I plan on visiting all eighty-eight on another heritage trip. Customarily, Japanese women do not show emotion, especially in public. Yet on my last day of the pilgrimage, at Zentsuji Temple, the seventy-fifth temple and birthplace of Kūkai Kōbō Daishi (the founder of Shingon Buddhism), something remarkable happened. Yuka, Yuki, and I all looked at one another and were immediately overcome with tears. Feelings of joy, sadness, and separation came upon us. Although we had only spent a few days together, I had learned so much and felt so bonded to them.

everyday osettai

In your daily life, osettai can take many forms. Osettai is a gift you give to the world through sharing what is most unique and honest about you. For me, it is my writing.

The author Marianne Williamson, who has given me a great gift with her words, encourages us to share our osettai with the world:

> *"Your playing small does not serve the world. There is nothing enlightened about shrinking so that other people won't feel insecure around you. We are all meant to shine, as children do. We were born to make manifest the glory of God that is within us. It's not just in some of us; it's in everyone. And as we let our own light shine, we unconsciously give other people permission to do the same. As we are liberated from our own fear, our presence automatically liberates others."*
>
> —MARIANNE WILLIAMSON, *A RETURN TO LOVE*

As I've discussed, my heritage and upbringing were different from those of many around me. But it is through these differences that I have come to see and appreciate how beautiful and unique we all are. No matter who we are or where we come from, every single person has a viewpoint that is theirs and theirs alone. Every one of us has something different to offer, with different talents we bring to the table. Remember that you—exactly how you are—are a gift. Share your truth with the world, as it is valuable.

Here are a few ways to practice osettai:

share your talents: Sharing your talent with others is a wonderful way to practice osettai. Host a workshop, coach a team, lend your skills, do a favor for a friend. Donate your crafts or your famous cuisine. If you're able to choose a career where you get to exercise your personal gifts, it will bring your life fulfillment. It may also point you toward your deeper purpose (known as *ikigai*) in the process. I can promise you, your life's calling will become clearer and more fulfilling when you become of service to others.

share your knowledge: As I've watched my mom do for my entire life, educating others is one of the greatest gifts you can offer. Teach a class, volunteer as a tutor. Knowledge empowers everyone, and the benefits are immeasurable. Or educate yourself! Why not enrich your life, right now, in this very moment? Sign up for that class you've always wanted to take or check out a book on a new-to-you subject.

share your home: As the people of Shikoku demonstrated, acts of hospitality bring joy to both the giver and the receiver. Host your friends or family for a home-cooked dinner, invite an out-of-town friend to stay with you, give someone a walking tour of your favorite neighborhood, or simply take a friend to experience your favorite local spot.

share your heart: Not all gifts can be seen; others can simply be felt. Just as one would offer a Shikoku pilgrim, share words of encouragement wherever you can. This can take the form of guidance or assistance to someone who is struggling, or it can be unprompted. Tell a colleague you think they're doing a great job, or thank your family members, roommate, or significant other for the things they do well.

This book is my *osettai,* my gift to you. When you are in need—if you are struggling, feeling stuck, experiencing heartache, or short on inspiration and light—I hope these words bring about a new way of thinking or living. I hope they will help create an opening for you, to inspire a new start where you embrace yourself and the unique story that has made you who you are.

As I said at the beginning, each of these practices is just that: a practice. They will help you continuously, and you will improve every day. But you're going to have to keep doing the work. These principles will serve you as golden repair during each and every part of your life.

Following the concept of *kaizen,* you may strive to always be better, but perfection will never be found. If you find yourself chasing perfection, I urge you to tuck that feeling away and stay the course. Remember the principle of *ganbatte*: Always do your best, but remember that your best is good enough.

Not only is perfection impossible, imperfection is beautiful in and of itself! Remember the philosophy of *wabi-sabi,* and look for beauty in unexpected places. Imperfection is the natural order of things—the fleeting nature of autumn, the changing color of the leaves, and, yes, the flaws in every human being.

If you find yourself in a tough spot but you cannot do anything to change it, *shikata ga nai!* Don't torture yourself over what cannot be helped. Stop, breathe, and let it go.

When you need someone to help pick you up, look to your *yuimaru*: those who make you feel good, those who have your best interests at heart, those who love you just as you are.

Be at peace with where you are on your journey. Practice *kansha*, and have gratitude for everything in your life—for the people, the experiences, and the opportunities.

Take good care of yourself. With proper self-care, you'll be better able to practice *gaman*, great resilience.

Above all else, see your life through the metaphor of *kintsugi*. Each and every one of us has times when we feel broken. Trust that your cracks will mend and make you even stronger than before. See these golden seams as the beautiful reminders of a life lived. Heal in your own way, move forward in your own time, and celebrate how everything you've experienced has brought you to this moment in your story.

You'll get to where you want to go. But in the meantime, trust that you're exactly where you're meant to be.

I wish you all the very best.

Ki o tsukete ne!

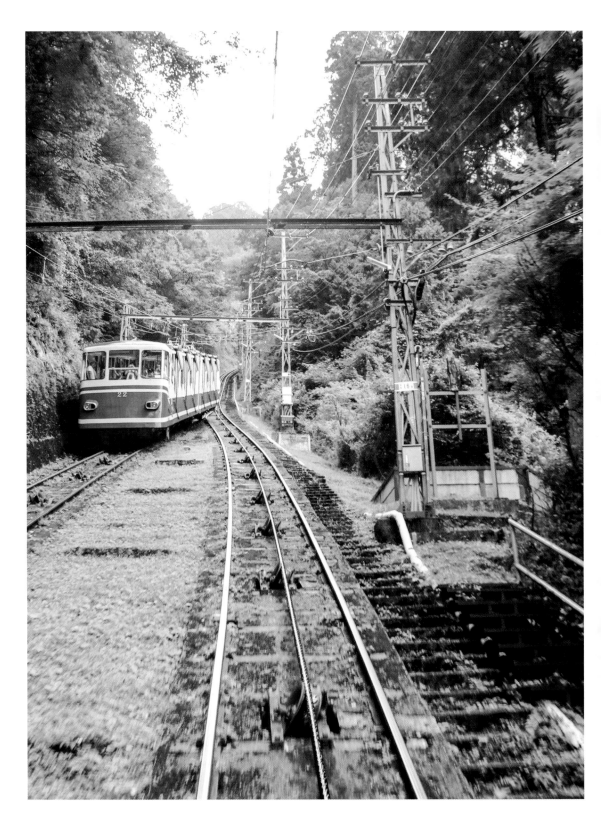

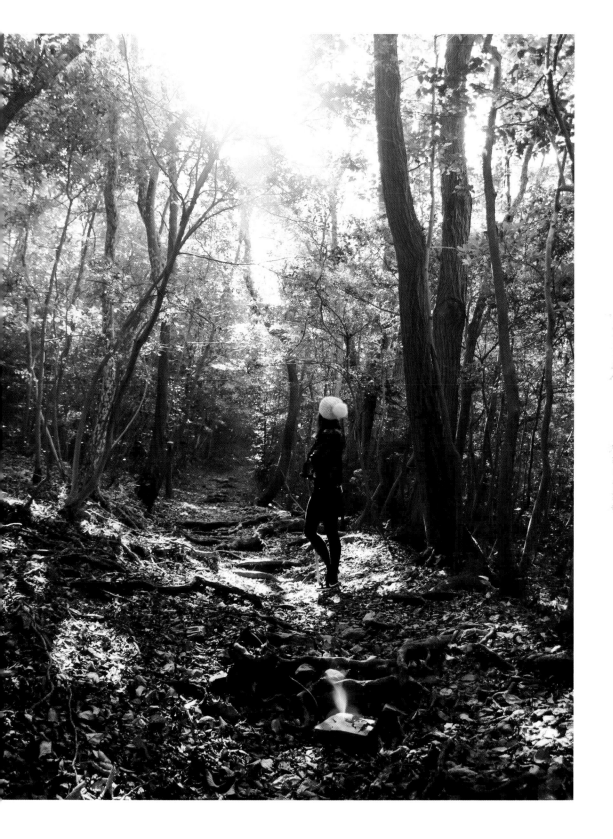

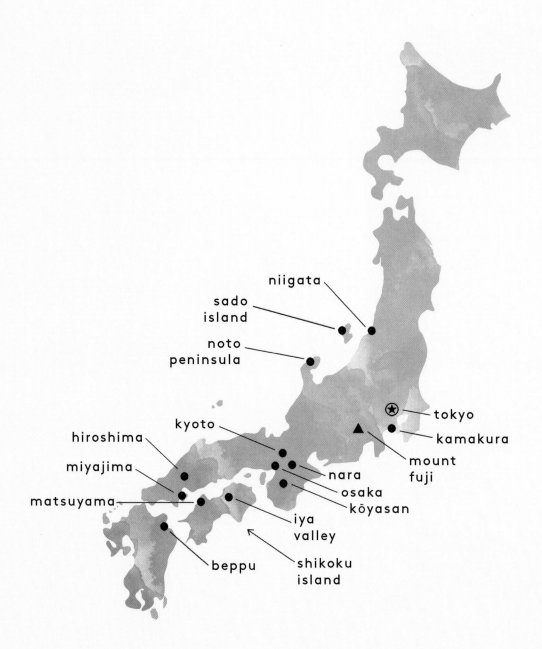

niigata

sado
island

noto
peninsula

tokyo

kamakura

kyoto

mount
fuji

hiroshima

miyajima

nara

matsuyama

osaka

kōyasan

iya
valley

beppu

shikoku
island

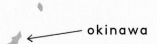 okinawa

explore
japan,
the land of
the rising sun
日本 旅，にほん たび
ninon tabi

THE LAND OF THE RISING SUN IS THE INSPIRATION FOR THIS BOOK AND THE PLACE WHERE MY STORY BEGINS AND ENDS, SO I COULDN'T RESIST SHARING MY FAVORITE JAPANESE TRAVEL DESTINATIONS. Though it's a small country, close to the size of California, there truly is so much to explore!

The changing seasons and vastly different terrains within Japan make it exciting to go any time of year—everywhere from Niigata in the north to the southernmost island of Okinawa. Hokkaido is up next for me, as well as the full eighty-eight temple pilgrimage in Shikoku. I hope to visit even more of the country over the course of my lifetime, to be reminded of the practice of kintsugi again and again, from the true masters.

kōyasan

Nestled deep in the mountains, surrounded by nature, temples, and radiating peace, Kōyasan is about two hours south of Osaka in Wakayama Prefecture. Life seemed to stop when I went to Kōyasan, a place where I could finally have a moment to myself. With its abundance of fresh air and serenity, Kōyasan tops my list of most magical places to visit in Japan, and even the world!

Years ago, my sister and I met up in Osaka, and from there traveled by car, train, and cable car to our first temple stay in Kōyasan. It was a bit cooler in temperature from the city, simply gorgeous, truly a dream.

Be sure to hike on the many historical trails and check out the wild hydrangeas when they bloom in midsummer. Pray, meditate as you walk through the Okunoin cemetery. Try the local shōjin ryōri cuisine (page 65), the devotional cuisine eaten by Buddhist monks considered sacred, simple, and in harmony with nature. I had the best walnut mochi (*kurumi-mochi*) in Kōyasan, and our meals at the temple where we stayed were some of the most memorable of my life.

Kōyasan is a holy place, a place to respect and cherish. I'd especially recommend looking into a temple stay, where you can participate in morning prayer sessions with the monks. At 6:00 a.m. each day, my big sister, Jenni, and I would wake to join the locals, monks, and other visitors in sacred ritual prayer. Because such a beautiful place is hard to keep a secret, visitors to Kōyasan have increased significantly, resulting in unprecedented crowds,

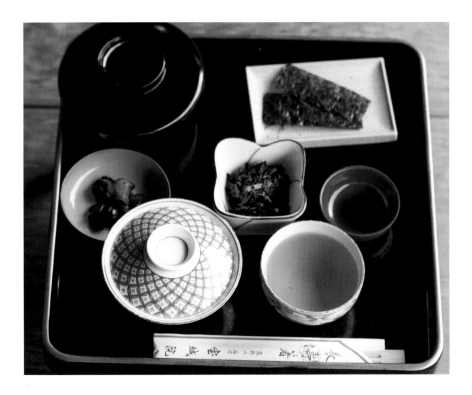

particularly during the spring and fall. Although most visitors are welcomed and are respectful of Kōyasan's history and cultural significance, there is growing concern that, should this trend continue, much of the atmosphere of peace and harmony will be lost. Kōyasan is a magical place I hope we can all show our children one day. My prayers for Kōyasan are that we continue to keep it peaceful, clean, and harmonious for many decades to come.

shikoku island

The least populated of Japan's four main islands, Shikoku has much to offer visitors, including gorgeous scenery, a Buddhist pilgrimage, delicious noodles, and some of the kindest, warmest people you'll meet in Japan. In Shikoku, the concepts of osettai and gaman are practiced every day! This is indeed the holy land, where I was educated on osettai as we made our way into the mountains and were welcomed with gifts and hospitality.

For many Japanese people, completing the 88 Temple "Ohenro" Pilgrimage is at the top of their bucket list. Walking the entire 750-mile path is not common; many walk a few days a year over holidays from work until they've completed the circuit. It is also common to wait until retirement and then take a week-long bus tour to make the journey. There are no rules here; simply showing up and starting to walk qualifies one to be a true Ohenro pilgrim.

The lovely women from Discover Shikoku, Yuki, Yuka, and my amazing guide Noda-san, taught me and my heart so much. I will never forget

Shikoku Island: My friends and mentors Noda-san and Yuki-san as we began our eighty-eight-temple journey! As we say in Japan, "Yoisho! よいしょ!"

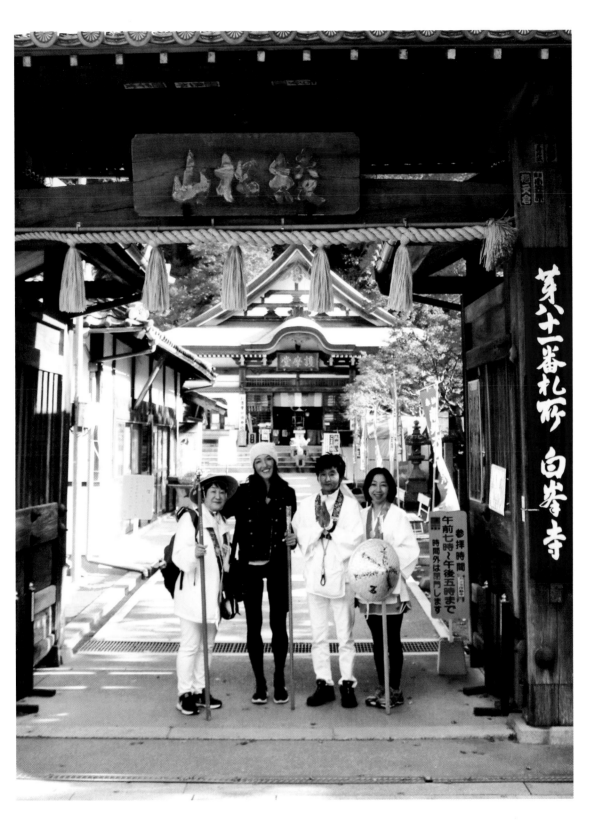

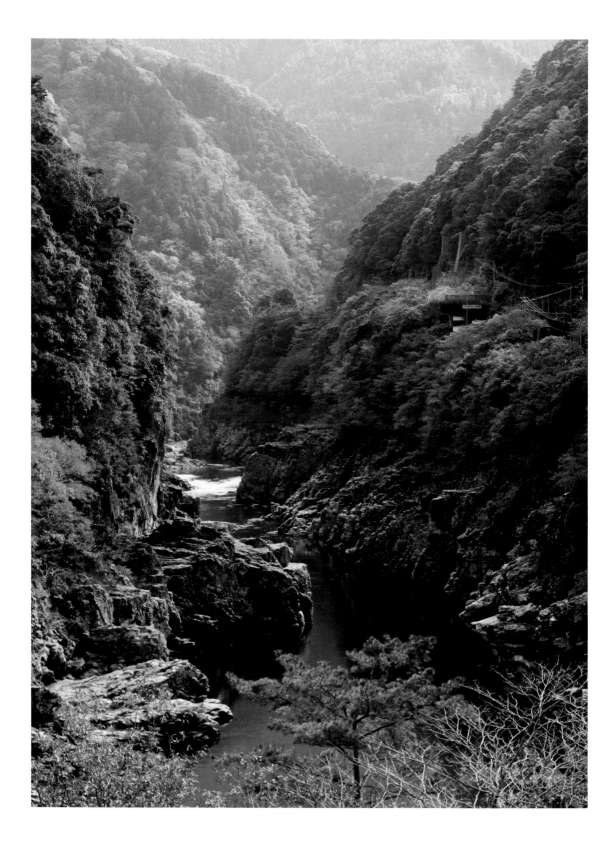

them as we laughed, cried, and hiked sections of the Shikoku Pilgrimage together.

iya valley

Located in central Tokushima Prefecture (part of Shikoku Island), this incredible hidden gem in Japan is not (yet) very well known to the American public. I found it to be the most naturally beautiful and peaceful of all the regions I visited.

I sampled delicious homemade soba and fried tofu, went for hikes, and snapped dozens of photos of this gorgeous valley that seems to have been forgotten by time. The locals I met took me on a tour to view their farmhouses on the steep hillsides where farmers must contend with the challenges of working on land more vertical than horizontal.

One highlight of my time in Iya Valley was seeing the village of dolls, where one woman has populated the once-thriving village with over three hundred life-size dolls memorializing her former neighbors, who have since moved to bigger cities or passed away. They appear to wait at the bus stop, run the local café, repair the electric lines, and attend the local schools. It's an incredibly touching experience highlighting the effects of population decline in Japan's remote countryside and it is impossible to observe with dry eyes.

matsuyama

Matsuyama is the capital of Ehime Prefecture and the largest city in Shikoku, yet maintains a quiet and relaxed vibe.

It's home to the famous Dōgo Onsen, a section of town known for its healing, restorative waters that flow through dozens of bathhouses and traditional inns, attracting visitors from all over the globe looking for a once-in-a-lifetime experience.

The local farmers harvest everything from rice to sweet potatoes, mikan to kumquats. This region has an extremely temperate climate and it's not uncommon to get two growing seasons for many of the main crops.

hiroshima

My solo trip to Hiroshima was one of my most memorable and emotional visits to Japan. My heart, my heritage, and the history of Japan and the U.S.—they are all deeply intertwined at Hiroshima. I came to learn and feel the past—the story of U.S. and Japan relations. As I toured the grounds of the Peace Memorial Museum, and saw the Genbaku Dome, the last building standing after the bombing, I reflected on the deep scars of the war.

I visited the original hospital grounds where the atomic bomb was dropped. I walked along the T-shaped bridge that was used as a target for the U.S. Army. I saw the watches and clocks at the museum that had stopped at 8:15 a.m. They are imprinted in my mind and heart. Visiting this site as a proud Japanese American was difficult, and emotionally charged, but it has always been part of my life's calling.

Hiroshima is steeped in devastating history, and the people there are some of the most resilient in the world; they look to the future while always honoring the past. They are masters at gaman. We have much to learn from them. I highly recommend going to visit Hiroshima to view a city that has overcome, and has become a living form of kintsugi.

miyajima

Miyajima, known as "Island of the Gods," is a magical place in the north-west area of Hiroshima Bay. The Itsukushima Shrine Torii, or floating gate, of Miyajima is stunning—during high tide, it appears to gracefully sit on the water, while during low tide it's accessible by foot. You'll be captivated by the scenery, the wild deer roaming around, the fresh seafood, and their memorable *momiji manju* (sweet local treats made with adzuki bean paste and a pancake-like crust).

Miyajima is a happy place, great for kids or to visit as a couple. I hope to head back soon to see the stunning historical torii gate in the water once again.

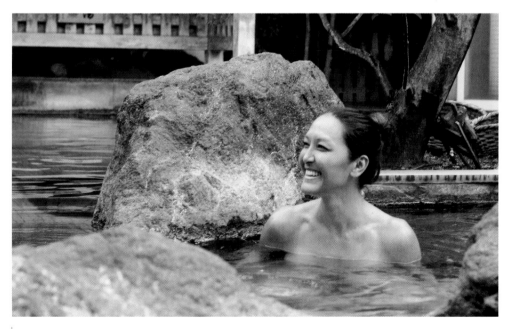

Beppu, Japan: Hot springs (onsen) are hands-down one of my top three favorite pastimes in Japan. Truly, the best way to relax and chill.

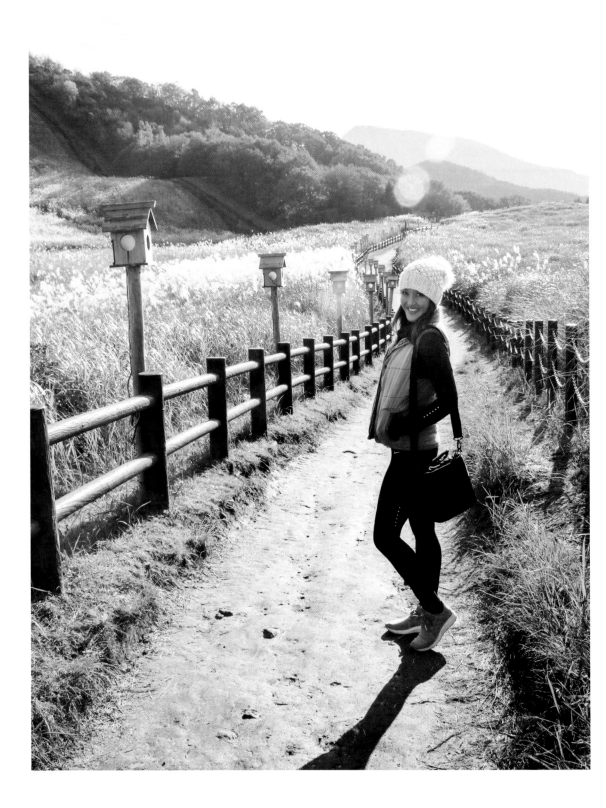

beppu

My mother's hometown and the place I call my second home in Japan, Beppu is located on the southernmost island of Kyūshū. Mom was born in Beppu in 1950, a place where you can still find homemade ramen, mochi, and senbei (crispy rice crackers), gorgeous parks, and, of course, the onsen (natural hot springs). It's the place where I first experienced hot springs, my Baachan's cooking, my grandfather's artwork, and my mother's true spirit.

There's everything from world-famous Kyūshū ramen (Mom takes us every year!) to homemade soba to the beautiful Beppu Bay and Takasaki-yama (the beloved mountain of monkeys!). I've been going there since I was five years old and still can't get enough of this small, adventurous, and beautiful hometown spot. Please visit and check out the local ramen (the spots in the alleyways are best), chill at the onsen all day, and just relax. We welcome you to come visit Beppu!

nara

Nara was once the capital of Japan, and many of Japan's oldest traditions originated there, such as the Japanese tea ceremony and sumō. A variety of different customs, materials, and practices were introduced to the Japanese via the Silk Road in Nara.

Located close to Kyoto, Nara offers so much to visitors. The people are welcoming, warm, and extremely proud of their land. I was able to visit during

Nara, Japan, a place that still captures the pure and traditional essence of Japan.

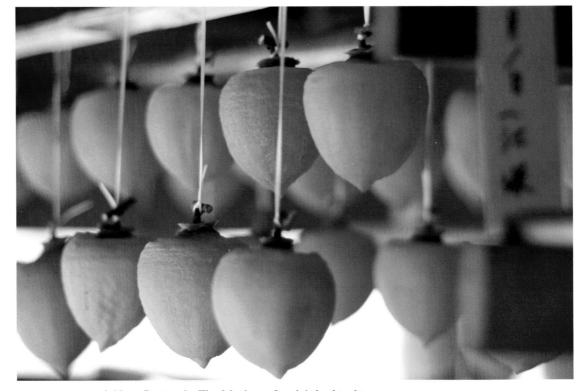

Noto Peninsula: The Maekawa family's *hoshigaki* persimmons, drying in the sun.

the fall and was captivated by the fields of golden grass (*susuki*), known as Soni Kōgen (Soni plateau). The most memorable meals I had were a Japanese nabe pot made with soy milk and fresh veggies, and a dinner of homemade soba noodles, hot broth, and local greens. Everything we ate here was a reminder of how to practice *eiyōshoku*—nourishing your body with intention. I was lucky enough to spend time in the company of a local baachan and try her delicious homemade rice crackers, treats, and tea in her home. I visited some nearby farmers and we harvested fresh greens together. On my most recent trip back to Nara, I was able to see the friendly deer, who roam the temples and are seen as "messengers of the gods."

noto peninsula

Off the main path and into the country, Noto sticks out from Ishikawa Prefecture into the Sea of Japan. Farming and fishing are the main industries, and the people living there still follow a traditional Japanese lifestyle as they've done for generations: farming, socializing within their local communities, praying at the neighborhood temples and shrines.

This is where I met Yamazaki Sensei and the memorable Maekawa family, who still dry persimmons (*hoshigaki*, locally known as *korogaki*) with love and passion for their craft. I will always remember my first time seeing korogaki being made by hand, the way that their family has practiced for centuries! I learned much from the people here—that hard work is never-ending (kaizen!), and if you find something you love, take pride in it.

okinawa

Referred to as a "blue zone" due to the robust health and longevity of its residents, Okinawa is located close to six-hundred miles south of Kyūshū. I was completely captivated by this magical, tropical island and its people, traditions, food. It's a place that has weathered an incredible amount of change through adaptation and resilience. The people of Okinawa are some of the most loving, open, hardworking, and happiest people I have ever met in my life.

The local cuisine is one of my favorites in the world. Okinawans cook with a surplus of brightly colored fruits and veggies. My favorites are imo (sweet potato), *gōya* (bitter gourd/melon), homemade tofu (this is the best in Okinawa, because it's lightly salted, and made fresh daily), the fresh, bright dragon fruit, and their miso paste, which has a distinctly different flavor than traditional Japanese miso.

I will always remember my Okinawan friends Mari and Hiromi, who showed us around their hometown of Tamagusuku. Tamagusuku, a small seaside town, is perfect for running and boating. Mari and her family have two delicious restaurants there: Hamabe no Chaya (浜辺の茶屋) and Yama no Chaya (山の茶屋).

You can also take day trips to the nearby islands of Ojima and Kudaka,

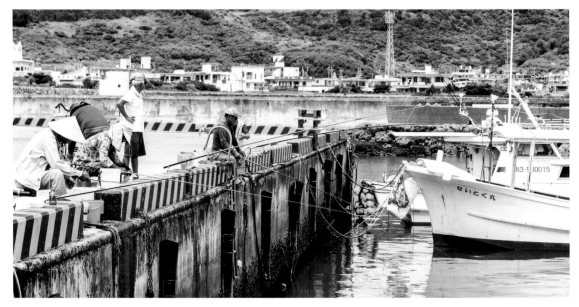

Okinawa, Japan: The locals here appreciate the simple life and their sunshine.

perfect for riding bikes in a totally secluded area.

There is a tremendous amount of U.S., Japanese, Okinawan, Korean, and Chinese history to learn in Okinawa. I recommend visiting Okinawa's Peace Memorial Park, as well as touring the caves where many locals sought refuge during the war.

Okinawa's lush scenery, gorgeous beaches, watercolor sunsets, friendly locals, and unique cuisine are unforgettable. Look for local artisans near the beach selling pottery and gifts.

I recommend flying into Naha, grabbing a rental car, and staying close to

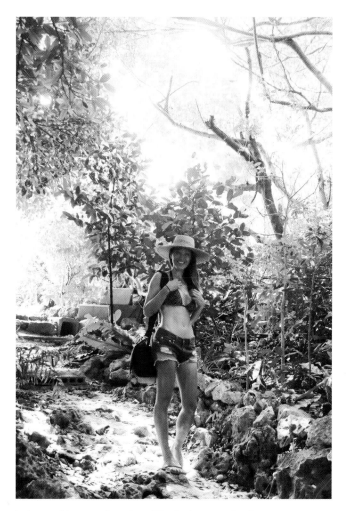

Some Okinawa beaches: The lush green landscapes are still unscathed and perfect for adventurous exploration.

Mibaru Beach, Tamagusuku, or Motobu Beach. Go explore off the beaten path with a friend or loved one. The beaches in some areas are still secluded and there's so much biking, swimming, fishing, snorkeling, hiking, and boating

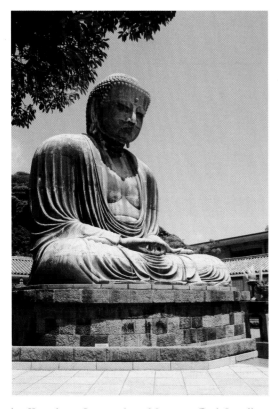

Kamakura, Japan, where Mom met Dad. It still brings tears to my eyes to think of their love story. Each time I am able to visit "The Great Buddha of Kamakura (Kōtoku)," I'm reminded of their first moments together. Such magic.

to be done! What makes Okinawa so memorable is its very special culture of resilience (gaman!) and the beautiful people.

osaka

After Tokyo, Osaka is Japan's second largest city and is best known for its diverse cuisine. Locals call it the "foodie's city," as its restaurants and variety of foods are much more concentrated than in Tokyo. The residents are bighearted and direct, speak their own dialect, and love to show off their hospitality. Be sure to check out Dōtonbori for food, shopping, nightlife, and exploration. Try the *takoyaki* (octopus balls!), okonomiyaki, local beer (I love Yebisu), *yakitori*, and udon noodles. Mom and I spent some quality time here together, trying out all the eats, and enjoying the nightlife and the local festivals. I will forever and always love Osaka for its memorable meals, shopping, and potential for getting lost and aimlessly exploring like any good tourist.

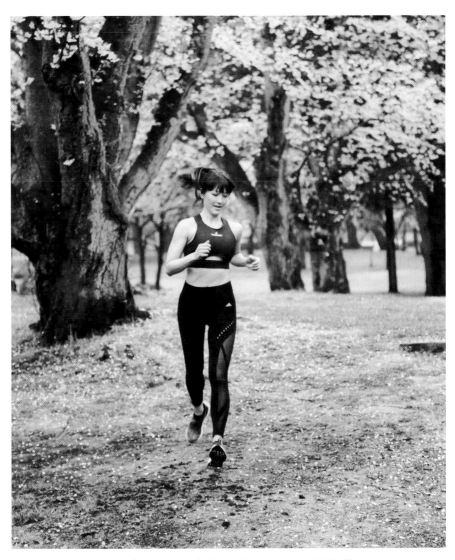

Beppu Park, a place where my whole family has experienced life. This park has taught me so many life lessons, from grief to celebration.

tokyo

When the wheels touch down in Tokyo, my heart always says, "You are home." I recommend seeing Meiji Shrine and Shibuya Crossing (Shibuya Scramble Crossing), grabbing sushi down a dark alleyway, eating as much tempura and mochi as you can find, drinking Japanese beer, and enjoying yakitori with the locals at an *izakaya* late at night. In Tokyo, you'll be close enough to see Mount Fuji and visit scenic Kamakura, the place where my mom and dad met at the Great Buddha. This place is sacred to me and to so many others who view its powerful offerings.

For the past six years, Mom and I have spent special bonding and research time together in Tokyo with her long-time college friends. We always purchase bento (lunch boxes) at the local *depachika* (department stores in Japan have a lower level that's full of delicious groceries! *Depa-chika* translates to "underground department stores") and then take the JR Yamanote line to Ueno Park, and enjoy our bentō in front of the Tokyo Metropolitan Art Museum where my grandfather's Impressionist paintings were once displayed. Tokyo is also where my mother attended university and became a school teacher in her early twenties. It was special to me to retrace my mom's footsteps with her in the city of her youth.

mount fuji

"Fuji-san," as the Japanese call it, is about one hour by *shinkansen* (bullet train) from Tokyo. Climbing season is short and crowded: July 1 to September 4, and the top can be cold and muddy, so come prepared! Research before you climb and, if you prefer, book a group climb and stay at a climber's hut when you get near the top.

I went to Mount Fuji solo, as a holy, healing experience. I packed my onigiri and water, wore my comfiest clothes, a headlamp at night, and gloves. I stayed in a mountain hut, which I highly recommend (you will have to reserve this hut in advance before your climb). I froze my buns off at the top, so be certain to bring more layers for up there! If you calculate it just right, you can watch the sunrise from the mountaintop. I felt very close to God in that moment.

Fuji-san is a UNESCO heritage site and an immensely popular destination for Japanese people and tourists alike. You can climb the whole mountain in one day or two depending on your skill level, but please ki o tsukete ne! (Be careful!) When you finish your climb, devour miso shiru, gohan, and tsukemono at the mountain base restaurants. Follow a bite with a trip to a local onsen to relax your achy muscles.

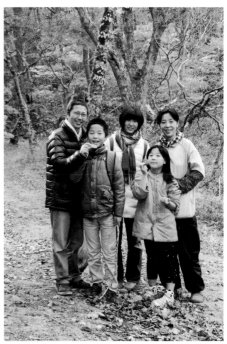

Chef Osaki-san and his incredible family hosted me on Sado Island. We foraged mushrooms all morning and cooked dinner for everyone in the evening.

sado island

Just off the west coast of Niigata lies Sado-gashima, a big infinity-shaped island populated by approximately 55,000 people.

My incredibly talented friend chef Kuniaki Osaki took me under his wing to gather local wild mushrooms with his

Sado Island boating. I mean, why not?

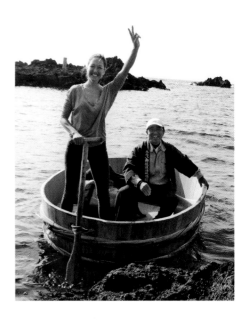

adventurous family during my last stay. Remember to forage only with an expert, as you want to be sure you're harvesting mushrooms that are safe to eat!

I did everything here: apple picking, persimmon harvesting, watching locals bake fresh Japanese banana bread, and forest bathing, followed by a lunch we cooked with my generous guide Fujiko. I got to spend time with some American teachers in the Japan Exchnage and Teaching program here, and see their curious perspectives on the quiet island of Sado. I will never forget the people of Sado—kind, polite, independent, and always graceful. They gave me many gifts I cherished: Sado rice, special Sado nuts, and the island's local sweetener. If you're looking for a peaceful and quiet destination, Sado is definitely one of the most laid-back places I've ever visited. I met so many special people on this trip and will never forget how welcome they made me feel. *Domo arigato*, Sado.

niigata

Niigata is known as "the sake prefecture," as it has the perfect climate for producing sake rice and is home to over ninety sake breweries! The local skiing in the winter is some of the best in the world, and I highly recommend hitting the slopes, followed by a hot onsen bath.

I only had a short time here, in the mountain town of Echigo-Yuzawa, but the locals were incredibly gracious hosts! We did some local research at a fascinating four-hundred-year-old tsukemono factory where they still do everything by hand like in the good ol' days! I stayed at a lovely old *ryokan* (inn) called Hatago Isen, which was conveniently located by the train station. The onsen, plus the local sake, was my favorite part at the end of our adventures in Niigata.

kyoto

After Nara and before Tokyo, Kyoto was the capital city of Japan for more than a millennium, from 794 to 1869. Kyoto is known for its many temples and shrines, classic architecture, geisha and maiko culture, and a passion for the traditional arts and kaiseki cuisine. Kyoto is full of wonderful hosts, and its people are rightfully proud of their beautiful city. A foodie could spend an entire day at Nishiki Market.

Kyoto is famous for its cherry blossom viewing, *hanami* in Japanese, as well as for its sacred and stunning temples and shrines.

Taste local Kyoto specialties like saikyō miso and *kitsune* udon and treasure Kyoto's local pottery, artisans, and stunning sunsets.

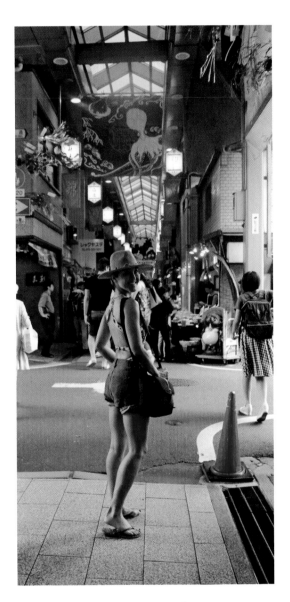

When in Kyoto, be sure to explore Nishiki Market as early in the morning as possible.

I must note, over the years, Kyoto has become much more crowded compared to the times I went there as a child. I still recommend doing the incredibly memorable Fushimi Inari Shrine (torii gate) hike, but I recommend going early or later in the day to avoid crowds.

A few of my other favorite stops are Kinkaku-ji (Temple of the Golden Pavilion), and Kiyomizu-dera Temple for its stunning views, and the shopping at Nishiki Market (in off-peak hours) shouldn't be missed.

And finally, Kyoto is where I first studied the sacred practice of kintsugi with Tsuyoshi-san, a highly skilled kintsugi artist.

You can still find some of the world's most precious pottery at Robert Yellin's Yakimono Gallery. And you will most certainly find the spirit of kintsugi and the magic of Kyoto all over this historical UNESCO heritage city.

The seed of everything I've talked about in this book was planted in Kyoto—a city very special to me for this reason.

a note from my mom

Dear friends,

Tomodachi no minasan,

ディア フレンズ ともだちの みなさん 友達の皆さん

Traditional Japan is changing rapidly, just the same as everywhere else in the world.

Open society, open world trade, open free speech. So many choices, so many changes . . . .

To a certain extent, the Japanese are losing their traditional ways. Perhaps we aren't as unique as we once were before.

But still, we are living in between the old and the new. The Japanese have tried to find a uniqueness in the fusion of cultures.

Before our unique Japanese culture fades away, please come and visit Japan.

We welcome you!

Sincerely,
Candice's Mom
キャンディスの母

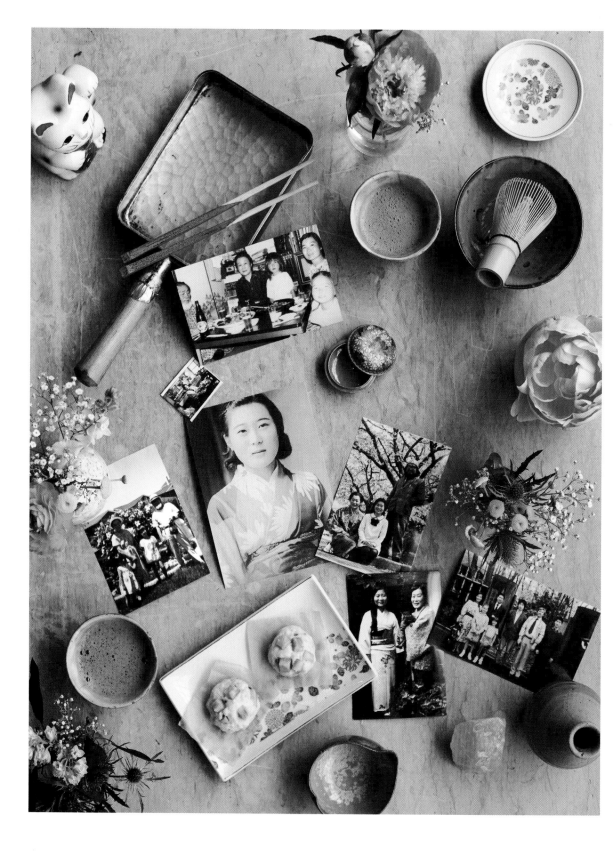

acknowledgments

ディア フレンズ 友達の皆さん. This book is for those whom I honor and owe a deep debt of gratitude. Thank you for being supportive, kind, and knowledgeable— *domo arigato gosaimashita!*

For Mom, you're an incredible example for us all. Thank you, Okaasan, for your humility, knowledge, and grace are what make you the world's Japanese sensei. You're the reason this book came to life. You're the heart behind the inspiration of Japan. On each page you helped me—thank you, this book is for you! **To Dad**, the most devout husband, dad, and humble guy. Thanks for being an example and hero for Jenni and me. Your open mind and selfless ways are why we devote our lives to others. **To Jenni**, this is us. You inspire me to stay loyal and confident; I look up to you. I honor our upbringing and thank you for all of your help in Japan! You are a guiding light to me.

To my Kumai 熊井 family, Takuko Nee chan (Takuko Kumai) 卓子 熊井, and the Tanaka family 田中 ファミリー , どうもありがとうございます, I'm grateful for the years we have spent together and the knowledge of our family's history and traditions. Domo!

To my Gwiazdowski family, Aunt Sally, Uncle John, Mikey, and the Casagrande fam, thank you for your undeniable support.

To the Inafuku family and Marie, thank you for sharing your family. To Yoshiko and Nobu, and Testsu-san, *domo arigato gosaimashita!* We are praying for Nobu's spirit.

To Hiromi Aoki and Ooike Isao Sensei in Okinawa, thank you for your time and sincere knowledge, I am grateful for all that you shared with Jenni and me in Okinawa!

To Yuki, Yuka, and Noda in Shikoku Island, to Osaki-san and your family, Fujiko and friends and Vy in Sado Island, I thank you! For my guides and locals in Iya Valley, Noto, Matsuyama, Hiroshima, Niigata, Sado, and all over Japan, *domo arigato!*

To the monks of Japan, **Kōyasan, Shikoku,** and beyond, I honor you and your light. Thank you.

To **Julie Will,** my editor who pushed me to do greater things. Thank you for pushing me to my limits and to the edge of the mountains of Japan, and for all of your hard work.

For **Karen Rinaldi,** thank you for your support, your knowledge, and your caring devotion to my work and to the country of Japan. I am so grateful to be publishing my work with you, Karen! *Domo arigato!*

For **Eve Attermann,** my literary agent to the stars; thank you, Eve, どうもありがとうございます for believing in my work—a true woman of grace.

For **Andy McNicol,** for showing me how to be strong, how to be a better author, and for being an example. Thank you, Andy.

To **these angels,** Christina Suarez, Constantina Konugres, Jade Rosenberg, Daniela Zamora, Rocky Owens, Olivia Boyce, Laryssa Loza, Kellyanne Rooney, Liz Lombardi, Candice Staley, Jen Batchelor, Cecilia Smith, I couldn't have done it without you and your devotion. You came into my life with passion and grace, and hardworking minds. Thank you!

To **my Japanese editors,** Miho Kumai Gwiazdowski, Saori Kurioka, Natsuko Aoki, Yukari Sakamoto, Natsuko Yamawaki, Yuki Kuzuhara:どうもありがとうございます! For your editorial knowledge, thank you, I honor our culture and your help has been valuable.

For **Lauren Scharf, my sensei, mentor, and friend,** I'm grateful, and owe a debt of gratitude to you for sharing our beloved Japan. A thank you to Mark Lakin for the intro!

To **Kazuhiro Yamazaki Sensei,** for sharing wisdom with me and all your students, I am grateful. I look forward to your emails, *domo arigato.*

To **Caroline Donofrio,** our edits and laughter make me smile. You're talented and such a gem, thank you.

For **Marcela Contreras,** I love you and your incredible art work! *Domo arigato.*

For **Sarah Haugen,** for your dedication and hard work, thank you. **For Bonni Leon-Berman,** thank you for the love and beautiful layouts!

For **Rona Tison** my mentor and sensei, thank you for teaching me what it is to be Japanese American. I'm proud to speak with you, and honor our heritage together. **For James Higa,** my mentor and sensei, for your mentorship. You're a light to so many of us with your humility and wisdom. *Domo arigato.*

To my WME IMG fam: My Justin, Eve, Andy, Scott, Julie, Googs, Jenni, Matty B, Rob, Bethany, Dave, Amir, a devotional thank-you for being my family for so long. Can't stop, won't stop.

To Strand Conover, my devout agent, you give me life/work, forever grateful. To Francesco Sersale and Taylor Rondestvedt, you are beyond the world, thank you!

To my Japanese culinary instructors: Elizabeth Andoh Sensei, Yukari Sakamoto, Mom, and my Great Auntie Takuko, thank you, I learn from only the best. **To the U.S.-Japan Council, Japan Society, Little Tokyo Service Center, and Morikami Museum**, thank you for preserving our heritage.

For my besties: Dana Hamilton, Courts Luni, Steph Areen, Michelle Halpern, Molly Sandman, Sajel Shah, Meredith Sherwood, my band of besties, I couldn't live without your love, life is fab and hilarious because of you.

To my *Well+Good* sisters, thank you, Liz Plosser, Emily Lawrence, Hannah Weintraub, Jordan Galloway, Molly, Rachel, Ella, Erin, Jenna—my devout gratitude!

To this incredible team of experts I'm honored to work with: Michelle Halpern, Hannah Kirshner, Dylan Going, Savannah Stark, Juli Akaneya, Robert Reyes, Sophie Solow, Eric Revilla, James Claytor, Carlos Garcia, Raul Santos, thank you for your hard work, I'm proud to know you!

To Jack Jeffries, your photography is magic, thank you. **To Kevin Kim**, devotionally, love your photos.

Carol Lee and Rebecca Grant: You've helped me in tremendous ways, especially with photo integrity, thank you!

For Bob Lange, Jill Smith, Marko Kuo; to Phil Gordon, Alex Davila, and Silva; thank you for being my support system and my family. I'm grateful for your hard teamwork! Thank you!

For my wellness sisters: Sarah Harvison, Sarah Merril, Natalie Uhling,

Rebecca Kennedy, Kathryn Budig, Vinti Bhatnagar, Rachel Ferrell, Jessamyn Stanley, Keri Glassman, Lee Holmes, and McKel Hill, and to my friends at the Maui Lulu Immersion, I support and love each of you, thank you.

To Yelena and Erica at Harper Wave PR, to the lives we inspire with your expertise, thank you!

To the girls: Christina, Andy, Tina, Suz, Alyssa, Molly Loven, Jenelle, Julie, Chrystal, Jess Bowman, Kristin Arnett, Indie Lee, Amy Duffey, Jess Morse, squad from Cali to NYC, I love you and thank you for being my friends for our years of growth. I honor our friendship.

To the boys in NYC: Barry Parasram, Brandon Trentham, Matt Paget, Akhtar Nawab, Marco Canora, Adam Rosante, Richard Rivero, Rocco DiSpirito, keep killing it.

To those I admire: Dr. Mehmet Oz, Arianna Huffington, Elizabeth Goodman, Michelle Promaulayko, Gabby Bernstein, Sophia Amoruso, Alexia Brue, Melisse Gelula, Marie Kondo, and Dan Buettner, thank you. I'm grateful for your contributions, for being prime examples for the world to follow.

To my friends: Ito En, Vitamix, Bob's Red Mill, Korin, MIYA, Marukan, ABC Carpet & Home, Eden Foods, Spectrum, Adidas, Madewell, Free People, Amour Vert, and Joie—*domo arigato*! Grateful for you.

To my loyal fans, I humbly thank you. You make me feel comfortable in sharing my story and my hope is you will do the same and share your story of kintsugi wellness with the world.

To the country and the people of Japan, to those who shared your heart and country: May you live knowing your heritage and traditions will be admired for centuries. Thank you for allowing me to study in Japan, for accepting me, for being an example, for being the gold standard. I promise to be truthful and to honor and pay respect to our Japanese heritage. *Ganbatte, ne. Ki o tsukete, ne.* **To the Universe God, those watching over me**, thank you for my blessings. I will continue to do your work for the people, with honesty, loyalty, and light. どうもありがとうございます. x ck

index

k i n t s u g i
金継ぎ
w e l l n e s s

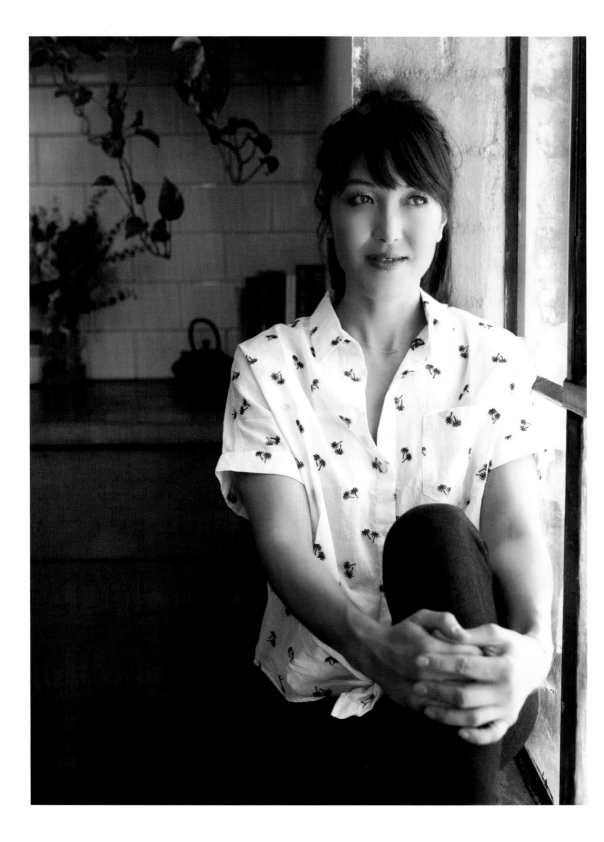

about the author

candice kumai is an internationally renowned wellness writer, chef, and content creator, described by *ELLE* magazine as "the golden girl of the wellness world." Candice sits on the Well+Good Council and was recently named one of Arianna Huffington's Top 20 New Role Models in 2017. She is a classically trained chef, wellness journalist, and five-time author of *Clean Green Eats, Clean Green Drinks, Pretty Delicious, Cook Yourself Sexy,* and *Cook Yourself Thin.* Candice contributes to wellness and lifestyle publications including *ELLE, Cosmopolitan, Bon Appétit, Shape, Girlboss, Men's Health,* the *Wall Street Journal, Forbes,* and *Well+Good.* A *Top Chef* alumna and a contributor on *The Dr. Oz Show,* Candice is a regular judge on Food Network's *Beat Bobby Flay* and *Iron Chef America.*

Instagram your love notes and your CK recipe pics @CandiceKumai. Get the latest at CandiceKumai.com.

HarperCollins books may be purchased for educational, business, or sales promotional use. For information, please email the Special Markets Department at SPsales@harpercollins.com.

FIRST EDITION

photographs by candice kumai unless otherwise credited

designed by bonni leon-berman

map, kimono fabric, and watercolor art by marcela contreras

Brief excerpt ["Your playing small does not serve the world… automatically liberates others."] from *A Return to Love* by Marianne Williamson. Copyright © 1992 by Marianne Williamson. Reprinted by permission of HarperCollins Publishers.

Library of Congress Cataloging-in-Publication Data has been applied for.
ISBN 978-0-06-266985-8

18 19 20 21 22   LSC   10 9 8 7 6 5 4 3 2 1

Images of Candice on pages 50, 165, 168, 172, and 318 by Jack Jeffries

Images of Candice on pages 10, 13, 28, 213, 230, 265, and 291 by Jenni Kumai Gwiazdowski

Images of Candice on pages 285 and 293 by Miho Kumai Gwiazdowski

Family images provided by George Gwiazdowski (mom and dad) and the Kumai and Gwiazdowski families